Mastering The Boards and Clinical Examinations In Internal Medicine

Hematology

A.B.R. Thomson

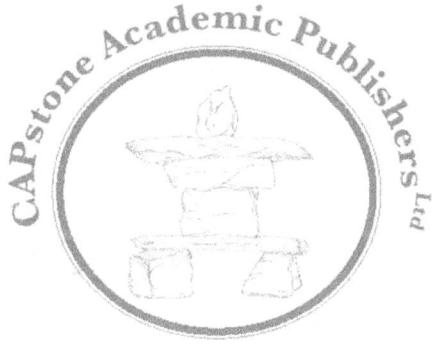

CAPstone (Canadian Academic Publishers Ltd) is a not-for-profit company dedicated to the use of the power of education for the betterment of all persons everywhere.

"The Democratization of Knowledge"

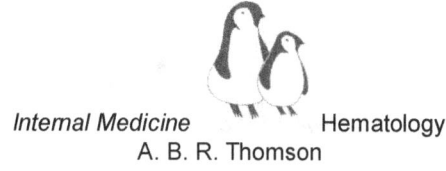

Internal Medicine   Hematology
A. B. R. Thomson

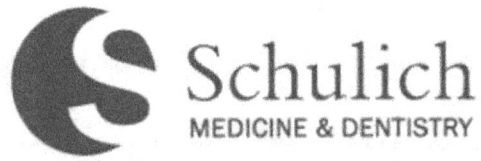 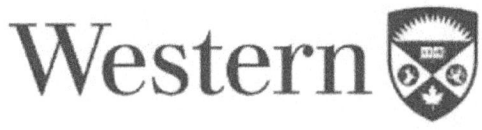

THE WESTERN WAY

Medical drawings by S. Lee and E. Howell

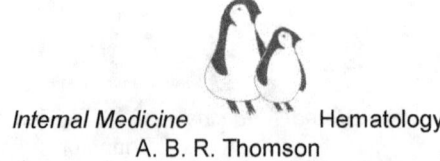

Internal Medicine   Hematology
A. B. R. Thomson

TABLE OF CONTENTS

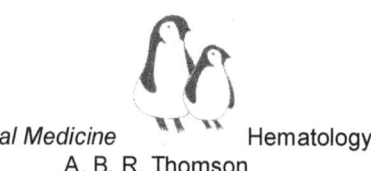

MASTERING THE BOARDS AND THE CANMED OBJECTIVES

Medical expert
The discussion of complex cases provides the participants with an opportunity to comment on additional focused history and physical examination. They would provide a complete and organized assessment. Participants are encouraged to identify key features, and they develop an approach to problem-solving.

The case discussions, as well as the discussion of cases around a diagnostic imaging, pathological or endoscopic base provides the means for the candidate to establish an appropriate management plan based on the best available evidence to clinical practice. Throughout, an attempt is made to develop strategies for diagnosis and development of clinical reasoning skills.

Communicator
The participants demonstrate their ability to communicate their knowledge, clinical findings, and management plan in a respectful, concise and interactive manner. When the participants play the role of examiners, they demonstrate their ability to listen actively and effectively, to ask questions in an open-ended manner, and to provide constructive, helpful feedback in a professional and non-intimidating manner.

Collaborator
The participants use the "you have a green consult card" technique of answering questions as fast as they are able, and then to interact with another health professional participant to move forward the discussion and problem solving. This helps the participants to build upon what they have already learned about the importance of collegial interaction.

Manager
The participants are provided with assignments in advance of the three day GI Practice Review. There is much work for them to complete before as well as afterwards, so they learn to manage their time effectively, and to complete the assigned tasks proficiently and on time. They learn to work in teams to achieve answers from small group participation, and then to share this with other small group participants through effective delegation of work. Some of the material they must access demands that they use information technology effectively to access information that will help to facilitate the delineation of adequately broad differential diagnoses, as well as rational and cost effective management plans.

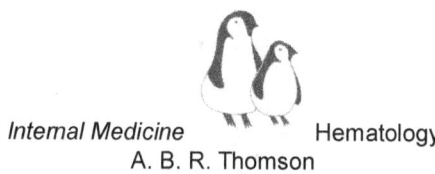

Internal Medicine   Hematology
A. B. R. Thomson

Health advocate
In the answering of the questions and case discussions, the participants are required to consider the risks, benefits, and costs and impacts of investigations and therapeutic alliances upon the patient and their loved ones.

Scholar
By committing to the pre- and post-study requirements, plus the intense three day active learning Practice Review with colleagues is a demonstration of commitment to personal education. Through the interactive nature of the discussions and the use of the "green consult card", they reinforce their previous learning of the importance of collaborating and helping one another to learn.

Professional
The participants are coached how to interact verbally in a professional setting, being straightforward, clear and helpful. They learn to be honest when they cannot answer questions, make a diagnosis, or advance a management plan. They learn how to deal with aggressive or demotivated colleagues, how to deal with knowledge deficits, how to speculate on a missing knowledge byte by using first principals and deductive reasoning. In a safe and supportive setting they learn to seek and accept advice, to acknowledge awareness of personal limitations, and to give and take 360° feedback.

Knowledge
The basic science aspects of gastroenterology are considered in adequate detail to understand the mechanisms of disease, and the basis of investigations and treatment. In this way, the participants respect the importance of an adequate foundation in basic sciences, the basics of the design of clinical research studies to provide an evidence-based approach, the designing of clinical research studies to provide an evidence-based approach, the relevance of their management plans being patient-focused, and the need to add "compassionate" to the Three C's of Medical Practice: competent, caring and compassionate.

"They may forget what you said, but they will never forget how you made them feel."

Carl W. Buechner, on teaching

"With competence, care for the patient. With compassion, care about the person."

Alan B. R. Thomson, on being a physician.

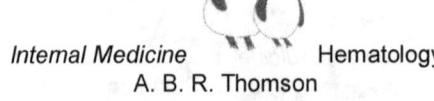

Internal Medicine　　Hematology
A. B. R. Thomson

PROLOGUE

HREs, better known as, High Risk Examinations. After what is often two decades of study, sacrifice, long hours, dedication, ambition and drive, we who have chosen Internal Medicine, and possibly through this a subspecialty, have a HRE, the [Boards] Royal College Examinations. We have been evaluated almost daily by the sadly subjective preceptor based assessments, and now we face the fierce, competitive, winner-take-all objective testing through multiple choice questions (MCQs), and for some the equally challenging OSCE, the objective standardized clinical examination. Well we know that in the real life of providing competent, caring and compassionate care as physicians, as internists, that a patient is neither a MCQ or an OSCE. These examinations are to be passed, a process with which we may not necessarily agree. Yet this is the game in which we have thus far invested over half of our youthful lives. So let us know the rules, follow the rules, work with the rules, and succeed. So that we may move on to do what we have been trained to do, do what we may long to do, care for our patients.

The process by which we study for clinical examinations is so is different than for the MCQs: not trivia, but an approach to the big picture, with thoughtful and reasoned deduction towards a diagnosis. Not looking for the answer before us, but understanding the subtle aspects of the directed history and focused physical examination, yielding an informed series of hypotheses, a differential diagnosis to direct investigations of the highly sophisticated laboratory and imaging procedures now available to those who can wait, or pay.

This book provides clinically relevant questions of the process of taking a history and performing a physical examination, with sections on Useful background, and where available, evidence-based performance characteristics of the rendering of our clinical skills. Just for fun are included "So you want to be a such-and-such specialist!" to remind us that one if the greatest strengths we can possess to survive in these times, is to smile and even to laugh at ourselves.

Sincerely,

Alan Thomson
Emeritus Distinguished University Professor, University of Alberta
Adjunct Professor, Western University

Internal Medicine   Hematology
A. B. R. Thomson

DEDICATION

To My Family

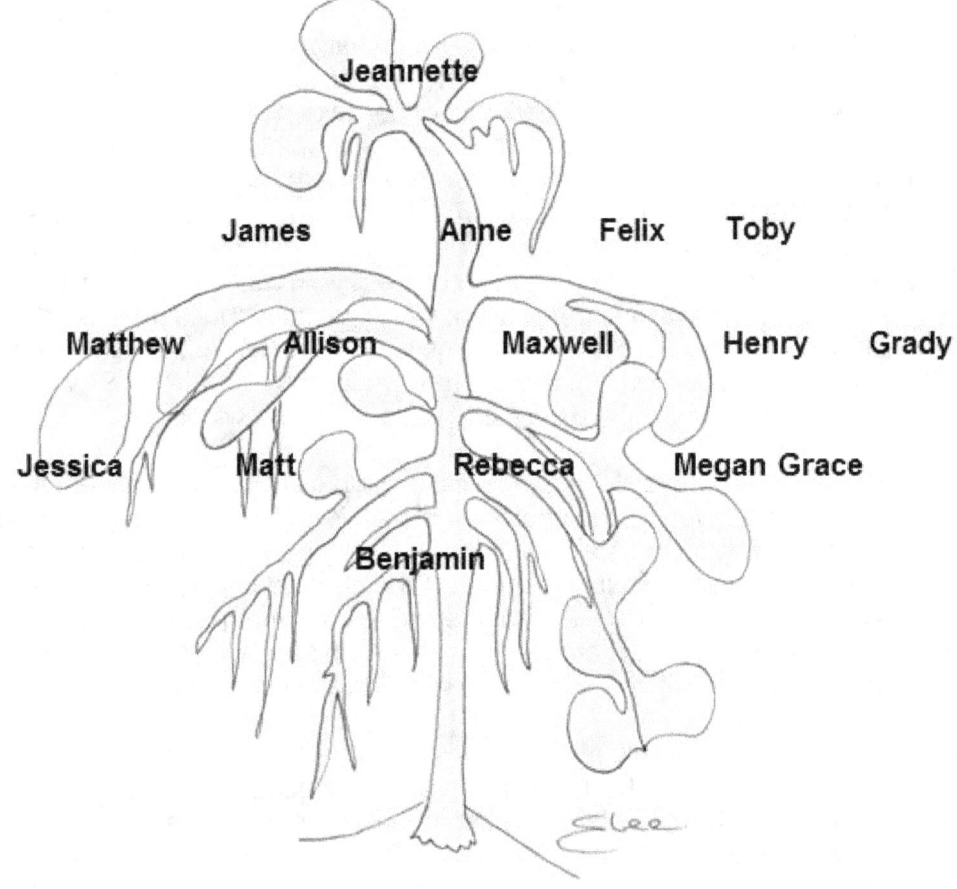

For your support, caring and love

During these challenging years

And always.

Mark 15:34

Luke 23:34

Domenichino 16:41

Corinthians 1:13

Internal Medicine   Hematology
A. B. R. Thomson

ACKNOWLEDGEMENTS

Patience and patients go hand in hand. So also does the interlocking of young and old, love and justice, equality and fairness. No author can have thoughts transformed into words, no teacher can make ideas become behaviour and wisdom and art, without those special people who turn our minds to the practical - of getting the job done!

Thank you, Naiyana and Duen for translating those terrible scribbles, called my handwriting, into the still magical legibility of the electronic age. Thank you, Sarah, for your creativity and hard work.

My most sincere and heartfelt thanks go to the excellent persons at JP Consulting, and CapStone Academic Publishers. Jessica, you are brilliant, dedicated and caring. Thank you.

When Rebecca, Maxwell, Megan Grace, Henry and Felix ask about their Grandad, I will depend on James and Anne, Matthew and Allison, Jessica and Matt, and Benjamin to be understanding and kind. For what I was trying to say and to do was to make my professional life focused on the three C's - competence, caring, and compassion - and to make my very private personal life dedicated to family - to you all.

Internal Medicine   Hematology
A. B. R. Thomson

Internal Medicine   Hematology
A. B. R. Thomson

DISCLAIMER

The primary purpose of this publication is education. The author, editor and publisher acknowledge that the development of new material opens to way for possible errors – what is correct today might not be the standard of care tomorrow. Readers are advised to ensure that the doses of drugs which they use are in compliance with their country's product information, and that the use of any therapeutic agent, be it a pharmaceutical or a technology, should be guided by local guidelines. There is often a wide diversity of professional opinion, and guidelines from one country are not always congruent with another.

The author, editor and publisher do not guarantee the safety, reliability, accuracy, completeness or usefulness of this material.

They disclaim any and all liability for damage and claims that may result from the use of information, publications, technologies, products, and for series provided in this publication.

We have made every attempt to trace the holders of copyright for material reproduced in this book. If by some oversight we have omitted a copyright holder, please contact us.

Thank you

Alan Thomson

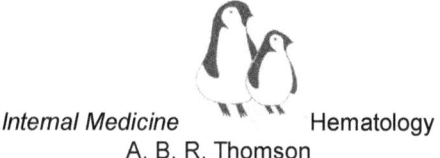

Internal Medicine   Hematology
A. B. R. Thomson

ARE YOU PREPARING FOR EXAMS IN GASTROENTEROLOGY AND HEPATOLOGY?

See the full range of examination preparation and review publications from CAPstone on Amazon.com

<u>Gastroenterology and Hepatology</u>

➤ First Principles of Gastroenterology and Hepatology in Adults and Children - Volume I – Gastroenterology (ISBN: 978-1494345624)

➤ First Principles of Gastroenterology and Hepatology in Adults and Children - Volume II - Hepatology and Paediatrics (ISBN: 978-1494345501)

➤ Medical Mini Review Series in Gastroenterology and Hepatology: Efficient Refresher for the Busy Clinical Gastroenterologist (ISBN: 978-1502472199)

➤ Medical Mini Review Series in Gastroenterology and Hepatology: Efficient Refresher for the Busy Clinical Gastroenterologist (ISBN: 978-1502472199)

➤ Practice Review in Gastroenterology (ISBN: 978-1500855321)

➤ Practice Review in Hepatopancreatobiliary Diseases and Nutrition (ISBN: 978-1500855734)

➤ Endoscopy and Diagnostic Imaging - Part I: Skin, Nail and Mouth Changes in GI Disease; Esophagus; Stomach; Small intestine; Pancreas (ISBN: 978-1477400579)

➤ Endoscopy and Diagnostic Imaging - Part II: Colon and Hepatobiliary (ISBN: 978-1477400654)

➤ Scientific Basis for Clinical Practice in Gastroenterology and Hepatology (ISBN: 978-1475226645)

➤ The Physiology and Pathophysiology of Gastrointestinal and Hepatopancreaticobiliary Disorders: Preparing for Professional Competence. (ISBN: 978-1500298265)

<u>General Internal Medicine</u>

➤ Achieving Excellence in the OSCE - Part One: Cardiology to Nephrology (ISBN: 978-1475283037)

➤ Achieving Excellence in the OSCE - Part Two: Neurology to Rheumatolgy (ISBN: 978-1475276978)

➤ Mastering the Boards and Clinical Examinations in Internal Medicine, Part I: Cardiology, Endocrinology, Gastroenterology, Hepatology and Nephrology (ISBN: 978-1461024842)

➤ Mastering The Boards and Clinical Examinations In Internal Medicine, part II: Neurology, Respirology and Rheumatology (ISBN: 978-1478392736)

➤ Bits and Bytes: Surviving Morning Rounds (ISBN: 978-1478295365)

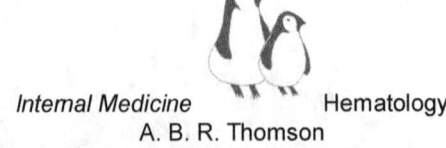

Internal Medicine   Hematology
A. B. R. Thomson

HEMATOLOGY

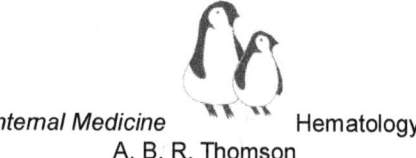

Internal Medicine   Hematology
A. B. R. Thomson

TOUGH TIMES FOR THOSE OF YOU WHO NEVER LIKED MATH!

- Sensitivity (sens)

  $$\frac{\text{True-positive test results}}{\text{True-positive plus false-negative results}}$$

  SN out: <u>S</u>ensitive test that is <u>N</u>egative rules <u>OUT</u> disease

- Specificity (spec)

  $$\frac{\text{True-negative test results}}{\text{True-negative plus false-positive}}$$

  SP in: <u>S</u>pecific test that is <u>P</u>ositive rules <u>IN</u> disease
  Note: The prevalence of disease does not affect sens or spec, and does not affect LR (likelihood ratio; please see below)

- PPV (positive predictive value)

  $$\frac{\text{True-positive test results}}{\text{All positive}}$$

  Given a positive test result probability the patient has the disease

- NPV (negative predictive value)

  $$\frac{\text{True-negative test results}}{\text{All negative}}$$

  Given a negative test result

  Note: ↑ prevalence of a disease → ↑
  prevalence → ↓ NPV

- When plotting the **ROC** (receiver operator characteristic) curve, plot sensitivity (true-positive rate, as the y-axis) vs. 1-specificity (false-positive rate)
  - The best cut-off point for optimal balance between sensitivity and specificity will be closest to upper left corner of this plot
  - Test with highest accuracy, Greatest **AUC** (area-under the curve) of the ROC graph

- **PLR** (positive likelihood ratio) = sens / 1- spec PLRs of 2, 5 and 10 ↑ probability of disease ~ 15%, 30%, 45%, respectively

- **NLR** (negative likelihood ratio) = 1- sens / spec

  NLR of 0.5, 0.2 and 0.1 ↓ probability of disease ~ 15%, 30%, 45%, respectively

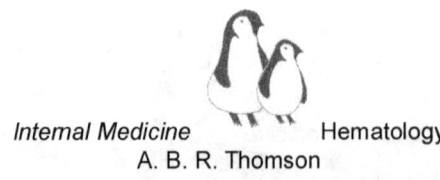

Note: PLR, NLR

- o Independent of prevalence of disease
- o Need to assess the pretest probability of having the disease
- o Risk estimates

	Outcome	
Treatment	Positive	Negative
Yes	A	b
No	C	d

ARR (absolute risk reduction) = [a / (a + b)] − [c / (c+d)]

RR (relative risk) = [a / (a + b)] − [(c / c+d)]

Usually, OR (odds ratio) can be substituted for RR or ~ RR

AR, RR, or are estimates of cumulative risk over time, usually at the end of the study

HR (hazard ratio) estimates the risk at a point in time (not cumulative, as is RR)

NNT (number needed to treat = 1 / ARR

"When you are transparent, there is no place to hide."

James Calvin

THROMBOTIC DISORDERS

To be considered here:

➢ Inherited thrombophilic conditions
   o Factor V Leiden (FVL)
   o Prothrombin G 20210 Gene Mutation (PGM)
   o Anti-thrombin deficiency
   o Protein C deficiency
   o Protein S deficiency
   o Dysfibrinogenemia

➢ Acquired thrombophilic conditions
   o Surgery
   o Trauma
   o Cancer
   o Anti-phospholipid syndrome (APS)

Inherited Thrombophilic Conditions

Thrombophilia

- Give the causes of inherited and acquired thrombophilias

   o Inherited thrombophilia
      - Prothrombin G20210A mutation
      - Anticoagulant deficiencies (Antithrombin, protein C, protein S)
      - Selected dysfibrinogenemia

   o Acquired Thombophilia
      - Immune
         ▪ Lupus anticoagulant or antiphopholipid antibody syndrome
      - Infiltration
         ▪ Solid organ malignancy
         ▪ Myeloproliferative diseases
      - Drugs
         ▪ Estrogens (oral contraceptives, hormone replacement therapy)
      - Pregnancy

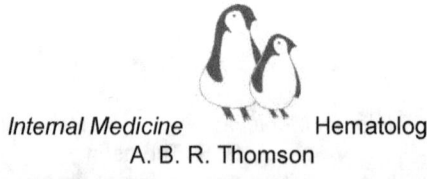

Internal Medicine   Hematology
A. B. R. Thomson

- Obesity
- Travel
- Trauma
  - Trauma
  - Postoperative state
- Senescence
- Idiopathic
  - Paroxysmal nocturnal hemoglobinuria (PNH)

- o Mixed Risk Factors
  - Hyperhomocysteinemia
  - Elevated levels of factors VII, IX, & XI

Adapted from: Ghosh AK. *Mayo Clinic Scientific Press* 2008, Table 11-19, 454.

- Give 5 conditions associated with thrombophilia and thrombosis.

  - o Common   -   Factor V Leiden
                        - Commonest inherited thrombophilia (in Caucasian)
                    -   Mutation of prothrombin gene
                    -   Anti-phospholipid syndrome

  - o Less common -   Protein C
                    -   Protein S
                    -   ↑ homocysteinemia
                    -   ↓ anti-thrombin

- Give the conditions under which testing for a thrombophilic disorder is appropriate and inappropriate.

  - o Appropriate   -   Idiopathic DVT
                         - First episode
                         - < 50 yrs
                     -   Recurrent DVT
                     -   Family history
                         - First-degree relative < 50 yr with history of idiopathic thrombosis

  - o Inappropriate -   Not fulfilling above "appropriate" indications
                     -   During an acute thrombotic event
                     -   < 2 wk after stopping anti-coagulation

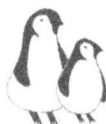

Internal Medicine   Hematology
A. B. R. Thomson

Useful background:

- Causes of purpura
    - ↓ platelets
        - marrow aplasia
    - abnormal vessel wall
        - Senile purpura
    - drugs
        - steroids
        - anticoagulants

- Vascular defects
    - Senile purpura
    - Steroid-induced purpura
    - Henoch-Schonlein purpura
    - Scurvy
    - Von Willebrand's disease
    - Uremia

- Coagulation defects
    - Hemophilia
    - Anticoagulants
    - Christmas disease

Adapted from: Baliga RR. *Saunders/Elsevier* 2007, page 391.

Factor V Leiden (FVL)

- Definition
    - The FVL mutation disrupts the first of three activated protein C (APC) cleavage sites, slowing the degradation of activated factor V (factor Va) and, ultimately, factor VIIIa", causing a marked increase heterozygotes and homozygotes in the risk of venous not arterial thromboembolism (VTE). (MKSAP 16, Hematology and Oncology, 2012, page 53).

    - Further ↑ risk

    - Combined heterozygosity (e.g., with PGM, prothrombin G20210A gene mutation)

    - OCP (oral contraceptive pill), and

    - Travel

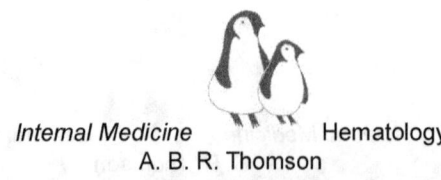

Internal Medicine   Hematology
A. B. R. Thomson

- Give the agents of choice to rapidly treat VTE in the post-operative state.

    - Normal renal function   -   IV LMWH (low molecular weight heparin; renal clearance)

    - Abnormal renal function   -   IV UFH (unfractionated heparin, RES (reticuloendothelial system) clearance

- Give the anti-coagulant used for long-term anti-coagulation of VTE.

    - Cancer   -   LMWH (low molecular weight heparin) for 3 mon or until cancer becomes inactive

    - No cancer   -   Warfarin

    - UFH (unfractionated heparin) is not recommended for long-term anti-coagulation in the patient with active cancer

Prothrombin G20210A GENE Mutation (PGM)

➢ Definition
   - "PGM stabilizes prothrombin mRNA, increasing prothrombin protein levels by 30% and 70% in heterozygotes and homozygotes .....", thereby increasing the risk of venous thrombolism (VTE) (MKSAP 16, Hematology and Oncology, 2012, page 53).

➢ Heterozygosity for both FVL plus PGM approximately triples the risk of VTA, and the risk is further increased by acquired / lifestyle factors

➢ Diagnosis
   - DNA

Anti-thrombin Deficiency

➢ Definition
   - Deficiency of thrombin, an ndognous anti-thrombotic protein, leads to reduced inhibition of serine proteases (e.g., thrombin, factor Xa), leading to ↑ risk of initial and recurrent VTE.

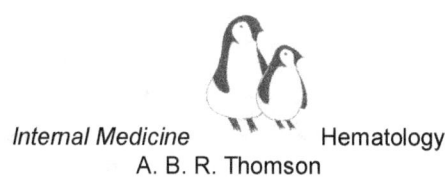

> Subtypes of ATD

Type of ATD	Mutation defect	Risk
I	↓ protein synthesis	High
IIa	Thrombin binding sites	
IIb	Heparin binding sites	Low

Protein C deficiency

> Definition
  o Deficiency of protein C, which is a serine protease that inactivates factors Va and VIIIa leading to ↑ risk of initial and recurrent VTE.

> Types

	Mutation	Effect of mutation
I	↓ protein C synthesis	↓ protein C activity ↓ protein C antigen
II	Altered protein function	↓↓↓ protein C activity ↓ protein C antigen

Protein S Deficiency

> Definition
  o Protein S deficiency leads to
    - ↓ degradation by protein C factors Va and VIIIa
    - ↓ inactivation of factors Xa by the inhibitor tissue factor pathway

Dysfibrinogenemia

> Definition
  o Mutations in the Aα, Bβ or gamma fibrinogen genes causing ↓↓↓ fibrinogen activity and ↓ fibrinogen antigen, resulting in ↑ risk of thrombosis and bleeding

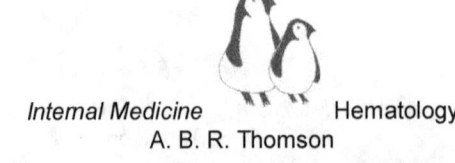

Internal Medicine　　　Hematology
A. B. R. Thomson

Acquired Thrombophilic Conditions

- ➢ Risks
  - o Surgery
    - ↑ risk of VTE
      - Outpatient   10x
      - Inpatient   70x
    - ↑ risk
      - Higher first 3 mon post-surgery
      - Persistent risk for 12 mon
    - Types of surgery
      - Orthopedic
      - Trauma
      - Cancer
  - o Benefit of prophylactic anti-coagulation
    - ↓ risk of VTE by 60%
  - o Trauma
    - ~60% develop DVT (deep vein thrombosis), 4% PE (pulmonary embolus), especially spinal cord or pelvic injury

  - o Cancer
    - Pathogenesis
      - Cancers may
    - Express tissue factor
    - Induce tissue factor by endothelial cells and monocytes
    - ↑ risk of VTE by 4- to 20- times
    - Risk highest with
      - Pancreatic and brain tumors
      - Metastatic disease
    - Continue anticoagulation for 3-6 mon, or until active disease is eradicated

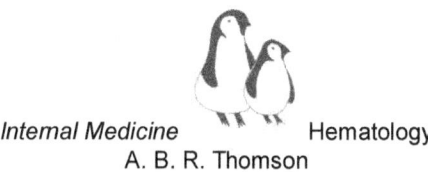

Anti-phospholipid Syndrome

- o Commonest acquired thrombophilia

➢ Definition
- o Primary or secondary autoimmune disorder characterized by the presence of antibodies against phospholipids or phospholipids proteins, and causing venous, arterial or microvascular thrombosis by
  - ↑ expression of tissue factor
  - ↑ activation of
    - Platelets
    - Complement cascade
  - ↓ function of protein C and anti-thrombin

➢ Pathogenesis
- o Antibody to B2-glycoprotein 1 bound to a phospholipid

➢ Clinical
- o Thrombosis
- o Pregnancy ↑morbidity
- o Skin necrosis within 5 days of starting warfarin
- o Venothrombolic, arteriothrombolic or microvascular embolus (disseminated microvascular thrombosis and multiorgan failure → catastrophic APS)
- o Adverse pregnancy outcome
  - ≥ 3 unexplaned, consecutive spontaneous abortions before week 10
  - ≥ 1 unexplained fetal deaths beyond week 10
  - ≥ 1 premature births before week 34 because of preeclampsia, eclampsia or placental insufficiency

➢ Laboratory
- o Lupus anti-coagulant
- o Antibody to cardiolipin (a phospholipid)
- o Antibody to B2 glycoprotein I (a phospholipid binding protein)

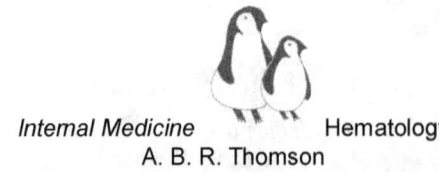

Internal Medicine　　　Hematology
A. B. R. Thomson

Please see standard Internal Medicine textbook, UpToDate, or current review such as MKSAP 16, Hematology and Oncology, 2012, Table 26, page 55 for details of diagnostic criteria for anti-phospholipid syndrome.

➢ Diagnosis
   ○ ≥ 1 clinical criteria
      - Vascular thrombosis, or
      - Pregnancy morbidity
   ○ ≥ 1 lab' criteria
      - Lupus anti-coagulant
      - Anti-cardiolipin antibody
      - Anti-B2-glycoprotein 1 antibody

• Give the criteria for diagnosis of anti-phospholipid syndrome.

   ○ Clinical
      - VTE or ATE (venous or arterial thromboembolism), or
      - Pregnancy morbidity ≥ first trimester miscarriage, or one fetal death

   ○ Laboratory
      - Dilute Russel viper venom time anti-cardiolipin antibody assay B2 glycoprotein I antibody assay ⎤ Positive on 2 occasions at least 12 weeks apart

➢ Treatment

A patient with an inherited thrombophilic disorder such as factor V Leiden, or an acquired thrombophilic disorder such as anti-phospholipid syndrome, is placed on long-term oral therapy with an anticoagulant. Within the first few days of receiving warfarin (especially high doses), skin necrosis develops.

• Give the pathogenesis of the skin necrosis which may occur when the patient with thrombophilia is given an oral anticoagulant such as warfarin.

   ○ An oral anticoagulant such as warfarin, especially when given in a high dose, will rapidly deplete protein C.
   ○ This rapid depletion of protein C causes a hypercoagulable state
   ○ The hypercoagulable state leads to thrombosis and skin necrosis

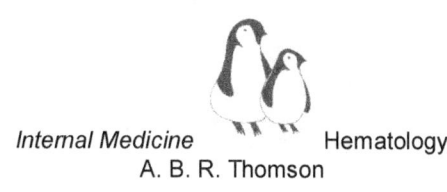

- o Initiate UFH / LMWH, with dose adjusted to level of anti-Xa if ↑aPTT
- o Maintain target INR of 2-3 using warfarin
- o For recurrent VTEE / ATE despite use of warfarin
  - LMWH, or
  - Fondaparinux

Abbreviations: aPTT, activated partial thromboplastin time; ATE, arteriothrombotic embolism; LMWH, low molecular weight heparin; UFH, unfractionated heparin; VTE, venothrombotic embolism

- o For catastrophic APS plus multiorgan failure
  - Resume anti-coagulation, if stopped
  - Corticosteroids, high dose
  - IVIG (intravenous immunoglobulin)
  - PE (plasma exchange)
  - Mortality ~ 50%, despite therapy above

Pregnancy

- Give the pathophysiology of the hypercoagulable state in pregnany.

  - o In pregnancy, there is
    - ↑ factor VIII activity
    - ↑ von Willebrand factor
    - ↑ Cyb binding protein
  - o The ↑ C4b binding protein results in more protein S that is bound, and less that is free
  - o The ↓ free protein S causes ↓ protein S activity, and thus ↑ coagulability

Acquired Thrombophilic Disorders in Other Diseases

- Give the laboratory changes in 4 conditions associated with acquired thrombophilic disorders.

	Anti-thrombin deficiency	Protein C deficiency	Protein S deficiency	Dysfibrinogenemia
Liver disease		+		
Nephrotic syndrome	+			
Pregnancy			+	
AC Rx		+		
Acute thrombosis		+		
Liver cancer				+

ACQUIRED COAGULATION FACTOR DEFCIENCY

- Give the causes of acquired coagulation factor deficiencies.

  - Vitamin K-dependent factors
    - Warfarin
    - Decreased nutritional intake or Malabsorption

  - Factor V
    - Myeloproliferative disease

  - Von Willebrand factor & factor VIII
    - Aquired von Willebrand syndrome

  - Factor X
    - Amyloid

  - Multiple factors
    - Liver failure
    - Disseminated intravascular coagulation (DIC)

Adapted from: Ghosh AK. *Mayo Clinic Scientific Press* 2008, page 450.

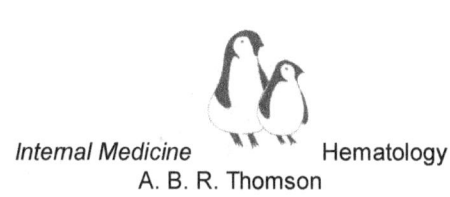

Internal Medicine   Hematology
A. B. R. Thomson

Vitamin K Deficiency

- o The vitamin K-dependent coagulation factors are II, VII, IX and X.

- o A malnourished patient with cirrhosis who is on maintenance antibiotic for prevention of SBP (spontaneous bacterial peritonitis) develops a pulmonary embolus.

VENOTHROMBOTIC EMBOLISM

D-dimer, DUS and Wells Score to Diagnose DVT

Step 1. Determine the diagnostic probability of DVT
Wells score ≤ 0 (low pretest probability)
↓
D-dimer → negative → DVT unlikely, no further testing
       → proximal duplex ultrasonography (DUS)
          CTA, or MRA
Abbreviations: CTA, CT angiography; DVT, deep venous thrombosis; MRA, MR angiography

For details on the Wells clinical deep venous thrombosis model, please see standard medical tests, or recent reviews such as MKSAP 16, Hematology and Oncology 2012, Table 28, page 57.

Anticoagulation Prophylaxis for venothrombotic embolism (VTE)

➢ Assess VTE for use of prophylaxis

- o Age   -   > 60 yr

- o CNS   -   NYHA class III / IV heart failure
- o Lung   -   Acute respiratory failure
                            -   History of VTE (venous thromboembolism)
- o Hematology   -   Thrombophilia
- o GI   -   IBD Inflammatory bowel disease)
- o MSK   -   Acute rheumatic disease
                            -   Immobility
- o Cancer   -   "Active" or being treated
- o Infection   -   Acute

- o Surgery

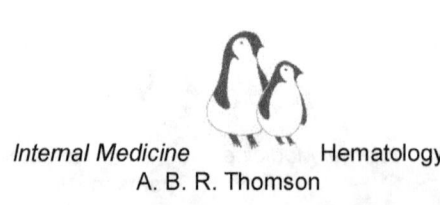

➢ Chose LMWH for
- o CVA
- o Active cancer
- o Surgery
- o Trauma

➢ Choose UFH
- o Renal failure (creatinine < 30 mL / min)

➢ Non-pharmaceutical options
- o Intermittent pneumatic devices
  - Prophylaxis indicated, but anti-coagulation contraindicated
- o VCF (vena cava filter)
- o Thrombolysis
  - Catheter
  - Directed pharmacomechanical
- o Surgical thrombectomy
  - For missing extremity thrombosis

➢ Stopping rules for warfarin

o	Usual practice	- At discharge from hospital
o	Hip arthroplasty / fracture surgery	- ~ 30 days post-op
o	Knee arthroplasty	- ~ 30 days
o	Abdominal / pelvic surgery	- ~ 30 days
o	Major trauma	- When inpatient rehabilitation completed

- There is a ↑ risk of recurrence of idiopathic VTE (50% in 10 yr). Give 2 factors which suggest that patients with idiopathic VTE require long-term anti-coagulation.
  - o ↑ D-dimer on / after anti-coagulation stopped
  - o Persistent thrombosis on DU (duplex ultrasound)

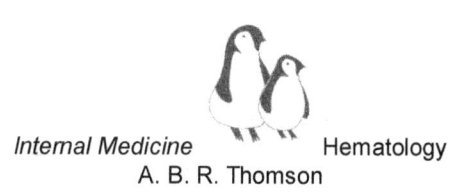

Internal Medicine   Hematology
A. B. R. Thomson

- Give the circumstance when a retrievable filter should be placed with a vena cava filter.
  - No likelihood for future anti-coagulation → no retrievable filter needed

---

A NEW TEACHING

Superficial vein thrombophlebitis → duplex ultrasonography

↓

  - Proximal greater saphenous vein thrombosis
  - > 5 cm superficial thrombosis

↓

  - Anti-coagulation, plus
  - NSAIDs, and
  - Compression stockings

CLINICAL GEM

- Give the safety of warfarin during pregnancy.
  - During the first trimester, do **not** give warfarin → embryopathy
  - For anti-coagulation for prophylaxis of VTE in pregnancy especially during the 1st trimester , use prophylactic or intermediate dose LMWH (low molecular weight heparin)

- Give the dose of warfarin to use to begin anti-coagulation.
  - Start with very low dose of warfarin, such as 1 mg/day

- ➢ Examples of drug interactions with warfarin
  - Direct gastrointestinal injury (e.g. non-steroidal anti-inflammatory drugs)
  - Altered gut vitamin K synthesis (e.g. antibiotics)
  - Altered warfarin metabolism (e.g. cotrimoxazole, metronidazole, fluconazole, amiodarone)
  - Interference with vitamin K cycle (e.g. acetaminophen)
  - Altered platelet function (e.g. acetylsalicylic acid, clopidogrel)

Source: Juurlink D. *CMAJ* 2007; 177: 369-371.

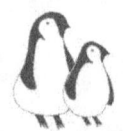

Anti-coagulant Drugs

Heparin

- ➢ Mechanism
    - o Binding of heparin to anti-thrombin → ↑ inhibition of activated serine proteases (e.g., Xa, thrombin)
    - o Metabolism UFN
        - - Degradation by
            - ▪ Endothelial cells
            - ▪ Macrophages
        - - Renal elimination
    - o Dosing based on weight
        - - Monitor aPTT
    - o LMWH (enoxaparin)
        - - Renal elimination
        - - T1/2 ~ 5 hr
    - o Weight-based dosing, with no need to follow aPTT
    - o Reversal protamine
        - - For UFH 1 mg / 1 mg UFH

Fondaparinux

- o Catalyzes anti-thrombin inhibition of factor Xa
- o Renal excretion
- o T1/2 ~ 18 hr
- o Reversal
    - - IV recombinant human factor VIIa

Warfarin
- o Mechanism of action
    - - ↓ hepatic vitamin K oxide reduction → ↓ synthesis of factor II, VII, IX and X, as well as proteins C and S
    - - Effect of vitamin K on oxide reductase is insufficient by cytochrome P-450 enzymes in the microsomes

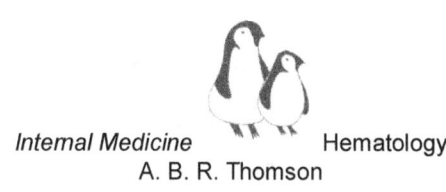

Internal Medicine　　Hematology
A. B. R. Thomson

- For a list of medications which ↑ or ↓ INR, refer to standard medical texts, UpToDate, or recent reviews such as MKSAP 16, Hematology and Oncology 2012, Table 30, page 58.

- Give the classes of drugs that interact with warfarin ("8 A's").

Drug or drug class	Risk of hemorrhage	Mechanism
o Antibiotics		
- Most agents, but especially co-trimoxazole, metronidazole, macrolides and fluoroquinolones	↑	- ↓ vitamin K synthesis - ↓ hepatic warfarin metabolism
- Rifampin	↓	- ↑ cytochrome P450 (CYP)
o Antifungals		
- Fluconazole, miconazole	↑	- ↓ CYP 2C9
o Antidepressants		
- Serotonergic agents (selective serotonin reuptake inhibitors [SSRIs])	↑	- ↓ primary hemostasis (may also inhibit CYP2C9)
o Antiplatelet agents		
- Acetylsalicylic acid, clopidogrel, ticlopidine	↑	- ↓ primary hemostasis
o Amiodarone	↑	- ↓ CYP 2C9
o Anti-inflammatory agents		
o All, including selective NSAIDs, Coxibs	↑	- ↑ mucosal injury - ↓ primary hemostasis
o Acetaminophen	↑	- ↓ vitamin K cycle
o Alternative remedies		
- *Ginko biloba*, dong quai, fenugreek, chamomile	↑	- Multiple, and often incompletely characterized
- St. John's wort	↓	- Multiple and often incompletely characterized

Adapted from: David N. J. *CMAJ* 2007;177(4):369-371, Table 1, page 370.

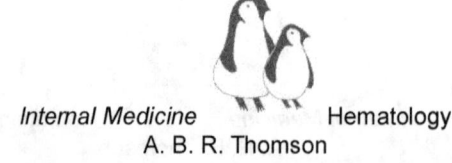

Internal Medicine   Hematology
A. B. R. Thomson

- Reversal of warfarin anti-coagulation in presence of life-threatening bleeding
  - Stop warfarin
  - IV vitamin K 10 mg over 1 hr, plus
  - FFP (fresh frozen plasma) IV, plus
  - PCCs (prothrombin complex concentrates), 3-factor PPCs plus FFR, or recombinant factor VII, or 4-factor PPCs

THROMBOCYTOPENIA

➢ Definition
- Platelet count < 150 x 10^9 / L (< 150,000 / µL)

➢ Causes: mechanisms
- ↓ production
  - Congenital
  - Nutritional deficiencies
  - Infection
  - Inflammation / autoimmune
  - Infiltration
  - Hematological malignancy
  - Hemolysis
  - Aplastic anemia
  - Myclodysplasia
  - Drugs
    - Alcohol
    - Chemotherapy
  - Falconi anemia

- ↑ destruction
  - Immune-mediated
  - Non-immune-mediated

- Splenic sequestration
  - Splenomegaly

➢ Clinical caution
- Platelet count
  - < 150,000 / µL (< 150 x 10^9 /L)   Thrombocytopenia
  - 30- to 40,000 / µL   ITP (idiopathic / immune thrombocytopenic purpura)
  - 20- to 50,000 / µL   ↑ risk of mucocutaneous bleeding
  - < 10,000 / µL   ↑ risk of intracranial bleeding

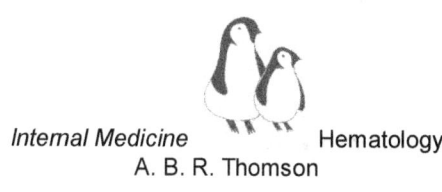

Internal Medicine   Hematology
A. B. R. Thomson

- Give the importance of platelet clumping in the patient with thrombocytopenia.

  o Clumping of platelets leads to the laboratory error in which the platelets in the clumps are not counted, leading to pseudothrombocytopenia.

Refractoriness to Platelet Transfusion

➢ Definition

  o Failure of platelet count to increase by > 10 x 10^9 / L (> 10,000 / μL) for each unit of platelets transfused

➢ Causes

  o Non-immune
  - Fever
  - DIC
  - Drugs

  o Immune
  - Alloimmunization

Abbreviations: DIC, disseminated intravascular coagulation

➢ Treatment

Pooled random donor unit of platelets

R ↓ ○

Single-donor, ABO-matched platelets

R ↓ ○

Access for possible HLA class I antigens

R ↓ ○

HLA antigens found

↙   OR   ↘

HLA-matched platelets   Crossed-matched compatible platelets

Ⓡ, refractoriness of platelet transfusion (failure of platelet count to increase by > 10 x 10^9 /L (> 10,000 / μL)

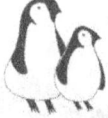

Internal Medicine   Hematology
A. B. R. Thomson

ITP (immune [aka "idiopathic"] thrombocytopenic purpura

➢ Definition

   o "…. an acquired autoimmune condition in which autoantibodies are directed against platelet surface proteins, leading to platelet destruction that may be only partially counteracted by increased bone marrow platelet production" (MKSAP 16, Hematology and Oncology, 2012, page 49).

   o ITP is a diagnosis of exclusion: for thrombocytopenia occurring in pregnancy, consider
- Gestational thrombocytopenia
- Preeclampsia
- HELLP
- DIC
- TTP

Abbreviations: HELLP, hemolysis elevated liver enzymes low platelet count; DIC, disseminated intravascular coagulation

➢ Causes

   o Ideopathic

   o Immune (e.g. SLE [systemic lupus erythematosus])

   o Infection (e.g., HIV)

   o Infiltration / lymphoproliferative malignancy

   o Iatrogenic
     Drugs

➢ Treatment

   o Indications
- Bleeding, or
- Platelets < 30-40,000 / µL

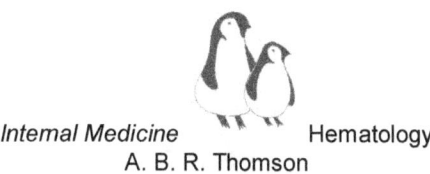

Internal Medicine   Hematology
A. B. R. Thomson

o Corticosteroids

- Dexaamethasone 40 mg/d for 4 days, then
- Prednisone / methylprednisolone 1-2 mg/kg per day
- IVIG (intravenous immunoglobulin), or
- Anti-D immune globulin, or
- Immunosuppression
- Rituximab, or

- MPM (mycophenolate mofetil)
  ↓ Failures

Stimulate thrombopoietin receptor to ↑ production in bone marrow megakaryocytes (delayed HIT)
  ↓
Splenectomy

HIT (Heparin-induced thrombocytopenia) and HITT (heparin-induced thrombocytopenia with thrombosis)

➤ Definition

  o 5 to 10 days after exposure to heparin, or at ≤ 1 day ↓ platelets if there has been prior heparin exposure within last 30 days (delayed HIT) risk of HIT is ↓ platelets by 50%, with individuals developing paradoxical arterial or venous thrombosis based upon their "4 T score" (thrombocytopenia, timing of platelet fall, now thrombosis (or skin necrosis or acute systemic reaction), presence of other possible causes of thrombocytopenia, and 4T score interpretation.

  o A platelet decrease of > 50% in a patient taking heparin or a thromboembolic event 5 to 10 days after starting heparin" (Board Basics 2013, page 158)
  o Late onset may occur up to 3 wk after stopping heparin
  o Recent exposure to heparin may accelerate HIT onset upon reexposure to heparin (serotonin release assay)

➢ Laboratory

More sensitive	More specific
○ ELISA measurement of antibody against heparin-platelet factor 4 complex	- C^{14} – serotonin release assay - Heparin-induced platelet aggregation assay

Abbreviation: ELISA, enzyme-linked immunosorbant assay

- ○ Process
  - Clinical suspicion

    ↓

- Calculate "4T" score if score high probability of HIT (6 to 8)

    ↓

- Sensitive lab test for HIT

➢ Diagnosis
  - ○ SRA (serotonin release assay) positive, but negative SRA does not exclude diagnosis
  - ○ Anti-PF4 / heparin antibodies (high risk of false positives, ↓ specificity)

➢ Treatment
  - ○ Stop heparin (do not use UFH [unfractionated heparin] or LMWH [low molecular weight heparin])
  - ○ In place of heparin, substitute non-heparin anti-coagulant
  - ○ Lepirudin (do <u>not</u> use in renal disease)
  - ○ Argatroban (do <u>not</u> use in Liver disease)
  - ○ Danaparoid
  - ○ Bivalrudin for acute cardiac interventions
  - ○ Do not use warfarin in place of heparin in HIT or HITT
  - ○ Continue anti-coagulation
    - Renal disease
    - No renal disease lepirudin, argatroban, danaparoid
    - Do not use lepirudin (renal excretion)

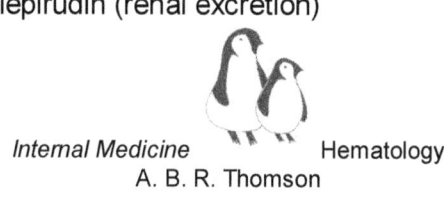

Internal Medicine　　　Hematology
A. B. R. Thomson

- o Stop heparin
- o Switch to non-heparin alternative anticoagulant, such as:
  - Danaparoid
  - Lepirudin
  - Argatrobin
  - Bivalrubin
    - Renal-dosing
    - Hepatic-dosing
    - Patient needing acute cardiac intervention

Thrombotic Thrombocytopenic Purpura (TTP)

➢ Definition
  - o An autoimmune disorder characterized by the development of antibodies against the protease ADAM TS13, leading to the accumulation of high molecular weight multimers of VWF (von Willebrand factor), which then causes abnormal platelet adhesion and activation, thrombocytopenia, microangioathic hemolytic anemia, as well as renal neurological and GI complications.
  - o Note the association with hemolytic uremic syndrome (HUS)

➢ Clinical
  - o Microangiopathic hemolytic anemia
    - Schistocytes, peripheral blood)
    - ↑ LDH (serum lactate dehydrogenase)
  - o Renal complications
    - ↑ creatinine
    - Hematuria
    - Proteinuria
  - o Neurological
    - Coma
    - Seizures
    - Stroke
  - o GI
    - Pancreatitis
  - o Associations
    - Pregnancy
    - HIV
    - HUS

➢ Laboratory (please see above definition)
  - o ↓ ADAM TS 13 activity and ↑ inhibitor titre suggest ↑ risk of relapse

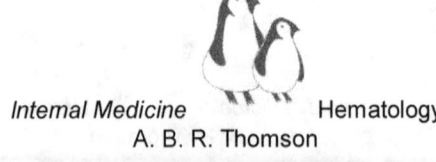

Internal Medicine   Hematology
A. B. R. Thomson

➤ Treatment
  o Potential life-threatening (10% mortality despite treatment)
  o Plasma exchange (PE)
  o FFP (fresh frozen plasma) transfusion if any delay starting PE, or if patient condition worsening
  o Role of corticosteroids not proven

Hemolytic Uremic Syndrome (HUS)

  o Overlaps with and very similar to TTP
    - E. coli O157:H7
    - Shigella
  o Differences between HUS and TTP
    - More renal than neurological complications
    - Often precipitated by infection
    - Associated with abnormalities in complement system

➤ Differential diagnosis of TTP-HUS
  o Malignant hypertension
  o HELLP syndrome / preeclampsia
  o APS (anti-phospholipid syndrome)
  o Scleroderma renal crisis

➤ Treatment
  o Because of the high mortality of TTP-HUS not diagnosed early and treated immediately with PE (plasma exchange), any patient with schistocytes in the peripheral blood, ↑ LDH and thrombocytopenia should be suspected as having TTP-HUS, and PE started.

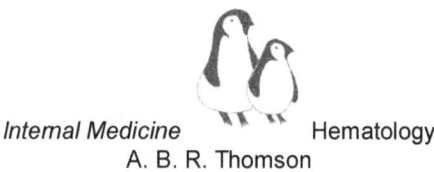

XX

SO YOU WANT TO BE A HEMATOLOGIST!

- In the setting of a patient with purpura, give the meaning of the Moschcowitz syndrome.

  o Speak English. Moschcowitz's syndrome is simply TTP (thrombotic thrombocytopenic purpura), an acute disorder characterized by:
    - Thrombocytopenic purpura
    - Microangiopathic hemolytic anemia
    - Transient and fluctuating neurological features
    - Fever
    - Renal impairment

Source: Baliga RR. *Saunders/Elsevier* 2007, page 391.

XXXXXXXXXXXXXXXXXXXXXXXXXXXXXXXXXXXXXXXXXXXXXXXXXXXXXXXXXXXXXX

DISORDERS OF PLATELET FUNCTION

  o Test for a defect in primary hemostasis when there is a personal / family history of mucocutaneous or post-surgical bleeding
  o Limited testing availability
    - PFA-100® (Platelet Function Analyzer – 100)
    - Bleeding time (BT)
  o ↑ BT
    - Platelet dysfunction
    - VWD (von Willebrand disease)
    - Thrombocytopenia and anemia
    - Abnormal vascular contractility

Thrombocythemia

  o Please see later description of essential thrombocythemia

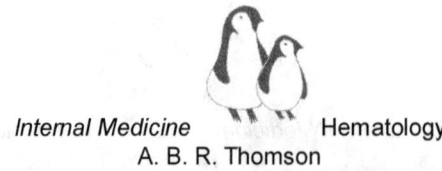

Internal Medicine Hematology
A. B. R. Thomson

Acquired Platelet Dysfunction

➤ Causes

- o Chronic renal disease
  - Treatment for acute bleeding
    - Desmopressin
    - Dialysis
    - Conjugated estrogens
- o MMD (myeloproliferative and myeodysplastic syndromes
  - Platelet transfusions
- o ASA / NSAIDs
- o Some foods e.g. garlic, ginseng

In the context of <u>thrombocytopenia</u>, there are <u>buzzwords</u> used on a MCQ which may be associated with the cause of the disorder.

- Give the likely cause of the thrombocytopenia when the following "buzzwords" are used.

Buzzwords	Suggested diagnosis on MCQ
o Schistocytes	– DIC (disseminated intravascular coagulopathy) – TTP-HUS (thrombotic thrombocytopenic purpura), aka hemolytic uremic syndrome – HELLP (hemolysis, elevated liver tests, low platelets)
o Teardrop-shaped RBCs	– Myeloplastic syndromes
o Hypersegmented neutrophils	– Deficiency of folate or cobalamin, causing thrombocytopenia
o Use or reuse of heparin o Thrombocytopenia plus thrombosis	– HIT (heparin-induced thrombocytopenia)
o Blood transfusion	– Post-transfusion purpura thrombocytopenia

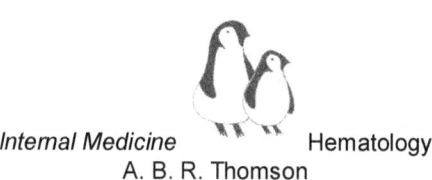

CLINICAL CLUES

A patient develops thrombocytopenia and purpura ≥ wk after a transfusion, or after pregnancy. You suspect post-transfusion thrombocytopenia.

- Give the method of diagnosis and treatment for post-transfusion thrombocytopenia.

    o Antibodies to HPA-1a (human platelet antigen) confirms the diagnosis
    o Treat with IV immune globulin

➢ Clinical

- Take a directed history of thrombocytopenia

    o Ideopathic

    o Dilutional
        – Massive transfusion/ infusion
        – Pregnancy

    o ↑ destruction
        – Autoimmune
        – Drugs induced
        – Connective tissue diseases
        – Consumptive (DIC)
        – Sepsis

    o ↓ production
        – Anaplastic anemia
        – Metastatic disease
        – Hematologic malignancies (marrow replacement)
        – Nutritional
            ▪ Vitamin B12 & folate deficiency
        – Viral infections (HIV, CMV, hepatitis)

Abbreviations: CMV, Cytomegalovirus; DIC, Disseminated intravascular coagulation; HIV, Human immunodeficiency virus

Adapted from: Ghosh AK. *Mayo Clinic Scientific Press* 2008, Table 11-17, page 452.

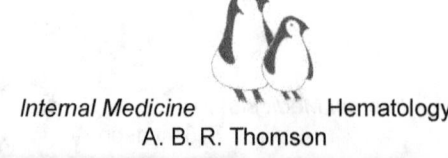

Internal Medicine   Hematology
A. B. R. Thomson

Thrombocytopenia in Pregnancy (aka Gestational Thrombocytopenia)

- o A "physiological" effect of pregnancy, due to
  - ↑ blood volume → dilutional thrombocytopenia
- o Suspect pathological cause of thrombocytopenia
  - If platelets < 50 x 10^9 / L (50,000 /µL
  - If ↓ platelets in T1 or T2 (first or second terms)
- o When platelet count falls in trimester 2/3, the diagnosis is usually gestational thrombocytopenia, preeclampsia, or HELLP.
- o These must be differentiated because early delivery is the treatment.
- o Other causes of thrombocytopenia are treated the same as in a non-pregnant patient.
  - – TTP-HUS
  - – ITP
  - – DIC

C	T1	T2	T3	Postpartum
	← TTP – HUS →		Preeclampsia	preeclampsia
	↓		↓ ~ 10%	
	MAHA		HELLP	
	Thrombocytopenia		AFLP	
	↓		↓	
	PE		Delivery	

Abbreviation: AFLP, acute fatty liver of pregnancy; C, conception; HELLP, hemolysis elevated liver enzymes low platelet count; HUS, hemolytic uremic syndrome; MAHA, microangiopathic hemolytic anemia; T, trimester; TTP, thrombotic thrombocytopenic purpura;

PT / aPTT	MAHA	↓ platelets	PT/aPTT	DIC	↓ BS	↑ SBP	Proteinuria	LE
Preeclampsia	-	-	-	-	-	+	+	↑
HELLP	+	+	N	-	-	+/-	+	+
TTP-HUS	+	+	-	-	-	-	-	-
AFLP	-	-	↑	+	+	-	-	↑

Abbreviations: AFLP, acute fatty liver of pregnancy; aPTT, activated partial thromboplastin time; BS, blood sugar; DIC, disseminated intravascular coagulation; HELLP, hemolysis elevated liver enzymes low platelet count; HUS, hemolytic uremic syndrome; MAHA, microangiopathic hemolytic anemia; PT, prothrombin time; TTP, thrombotic thrombocytopenic purpura

---

CLINICAL CLUES
- o Preeclampsia
    - Half occur T3, ~ half post-partum
    - 10% progress to HELLP
- o HELLP
    - Half have hypertension
    - Half are normotensive

➤ Treatment target
- o When to give platelets in pregnancy
    - Asymptomatic, Pl < 50,000 / µL
    - Symptomatic, < 30 – 40,000 / µL
    - Cesarean section, < 50,000 / µL
    - Neuraxial anesthesia, < 80,000 / µL
- o Thrombocytopenia in neonate
    - Anti-platelet antibodies may cross the placenta
    - Thrombocytopenia in neonate ~ 10%
    - Problems with measuring fetal platelet levels
        - Scalp vein sampling is misleading
        - Umbilical cord sampling may cause miscarriage (1%)

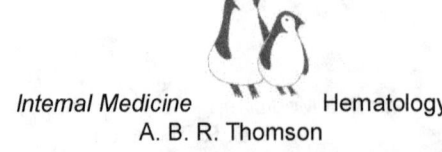

BLEEDING DISORDERS

```
CLINICAL GEMS AND PEARLS
Commonest causes
    o  ↑ PT             -  Vitamin K deficiency, including warfarin
                        -  Liver disease
                        -  DIC
                        -  Factor VII deficiency, acquired
    o  ↑aPTT            -  Lupus inhibitor
                        -  Hemophilia

•  Give the reason why the citrate-containing tubes must be filled at
   phlebotomy.
    o  Less than complete filling of the collection tubes results in an excess of
       citrate for the volume of plasma, and the PT and aPTT will be falsely high.

Abbreviation: PT, prothrombin time; aPTT, active partial thromboplastin time
```

➢ Classification

The classification of congenital and acquired disorders of coagulation is beyond the scope of this book. The interested reader is referred to standard textbooks of Hematology, or the reviews such as MKSAP 16, Hematology, 2012, Table 22 pages 44-45.

• Give a simple classification of bleeding disorders.

o Primary	– Formation of platelet plus at site of vascular damage
	– Failure
	▪ Bleeding gums, nose
	▪ Easy bruising
	▪ Menorrhea
o Secondary	– The coagulation cascade begins when the site of vascular damage is expressed
	- Failure
	▪ Bleeding into muscles, joints
	▪ Delayed bleeding

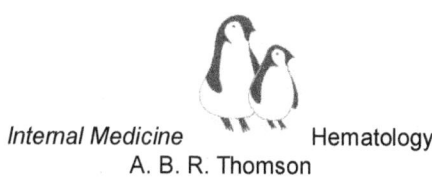

Internal Medicine   Hematology
A. B. R. Thomson

o Failure of primary or secondary hemostasis → bleeding after
  - Surgery
  - Trauma
  - Childbirth

➤ Laboratory

- In the patient with both ↑ PT and ↑ aPTT, give the role of the thrombin clotting (TCT).

  o To determine if there is
    - A thrombin inhibitor (e.g. heparin)
    - Hypo-/dysfibrinogenemia

- Give the interpretation of a mixing study performed when there is ↑ aPTT.

  o Correction of aPTT with adding normal plasma
    - Factor deficiency
  o Incomplete correction of aPTT
    - Presence of an inhibitor

- Give the diagnostic methods used to identify a bleeding disorder.
  o PT

  o aPTT

  o Mixing study
    - Mix plasma from patient with normal plasma to differentiate deficiency vs. inhibitor of factors
    - Mixing study
      ▪ Correct → factor deficiency
      ▪ Does not correct → circulating (inhibitor) anticoagulant
  o Bleeding time
    - Platelet disorders
    - Integrity of vessel walls
  o Thrombin time tests
    - Fibrinogen → fibrin conversion
  o Fibrinogen, fibrinogen degradation product, D-dimer test
    - ↑ fibrinolysis

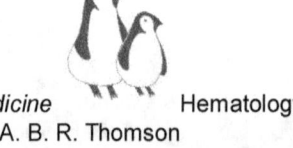

- Give the PT, aPTT and result of mixing studies of the following coagulation disorders.

Coagulation test		Mixing study corrects	Abnormality Deficiency
PT	aPTT		
↑	↑		Single or multiple
↑	N		VII
N	↑	Yes	VIII, IX, XI, XII
			XII without bleeding
N	↑	No	Circulating inhibitor (anticoagulant) – think of conditions such as SLE
N	N / ↑		Think of VWD

Note: the expected changes with therapeutic anti-coagulation

- Give the effect of treatment (Rx) with warfarin and UFH on the PT, aPTT and mixing study correction.

Rx	PT	aPTT	Mixing study correction
o Warfarin	↑↑	↑	
o UFH	N	↑	Yes

Abbreviations: aPTT, partial thromboplastin time; N, normal; PT, prothrombin time; SLE, systemic erythematosus; UFH, unfractioned heparin; VWD, Von Willebrand disease

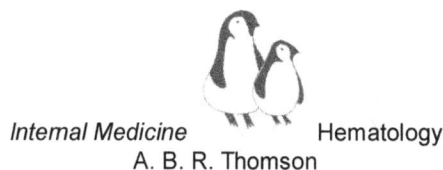

Hemophilia A and B

➢ Definition

   o X-linked recessive disorders due to deficiency of factor VIII (hemophilia) or factor IX (hemophilia B)

➢ Clinical

   o Hemarthrosis → joint degeneration

   o CNS bleeding

   o Bleeding after
   - Surgery
   - Trauma

   o X-linked disorders

Hemophilia	Factor Deficiency
A	VIII
B	IX

➢ Diagnosis

   o Normal, aPTT ↑, corrects with addition of normal plasma (mixing study) assess for HCV, HIV (from transfusion > 25 yr ago)

➢ Therapy

   o Transfusion as needed for bleeding

   o Factor replacement
   - VIII A
   - IX B
   - Consider prophylactic therapy (↓ arthropathy)

   o Acute bleeding   ⎤ Desmopressin
   o Prophylaxis for minor procedures   ⎦

   o IV concentrates of factor VII or IX

   o Desmopressin

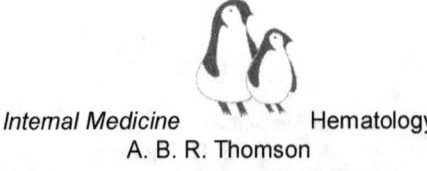

Internal Medicine   Hematology
A. B. R. Thomson

XXX

SO YOU WANT TO BE A HEMATOLOGIST!

In the patient with hemophilia A, diabetics, hypertension, dyslipoproteinemia, and who smokes, and has had a previous TIA, give the recommended dose of aspirin to use prophylactically.

- o Fooled you! Maybe? Correct answer is NO ASA or NSAIDs in hemophilia A or B
- o Say it again
- o ASA and NSAIDs are contraindicated in persons with hemophilia

XXXXXXXXXXXXXXXXXXXXXXXXXXXXXXXXXXXXXXXXXXXXXXXXXXXXXXXXXXX

THERAPEUTIC CAUTION

- Give the dose of ASA (aspirin) to be used for cardiovascular protection in the patient with hemophilia.

  - o Ouch! ASA is contraindicated in hemophilia.

Acquired Hemophilia

➤ Definition
  - o An acquired reduction in factor VIII from an inhibitor, resulting in multifocal mucocutaneous bleeding (not hemarthroses)

➤ Associations
  - o Postpartum
  - o Autoimmune
  - o Malignancy
  - o Ideopathic (50%)

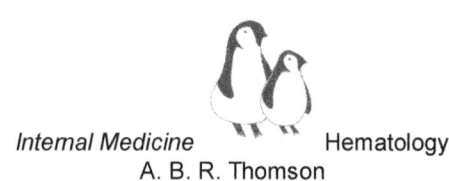

Internal Medicine   Hematology
A. B. R. Thomson

- ➢ Laboratory findings
  - o ↓ factor VIII
  - o Non-correction on mixing study (i.e., presence of an inhibitor)

- ➢ Treatment
  - o < 5 Bethesda units factor VIII concentrates
  - o > 5 Bethesda units
    - Rh (recombinant human) VIIa concentrate, or
    - Prothrombin complex (to activate factor X and intrinsic pathway

Liver Disease and Coagulopathy

- ➢ Pathogenesis
  - o Coagulopathy
    - ↓ D-dimer clearance
  - o Hypo- / dysfibrinogenemia
    - ↓ fibrinogen
    - ↑ fibrinolysis
  - o Thrombocytopenia
    - Hypersplenism
    - ↑ platelet clearance
    - May be refractory to platelet transfusion

- ➢ Laboratory
  - o ↑ PT
  - o ↑ aPTT
  - o ↑ TCT
  - o ↓ platelets
  - o ↓ fibrinogen concentration and function
  - o ↑ D-dimer

- ➢ Treatment
  - o Treat underlying liver disease
  - o FFP plus vitamin K

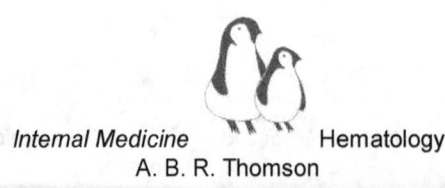

Disseminated Intravacular Coagulation (DIC)

➢ Pathogenesis
  o Production of normal thrombin leads to
    - ↑ consumption of clotting factors and platelets
    - ↑ fibrinolysis

➢ Causes / associations

• Give the causes of DIC.

  o Infection
    - Infection or sepsis (bacterial)
  o Infiltration
    - Malignancies (hematologic & solid organs)
    - Solid tumors
  o Drugs/ toxins
    - Snake bite
  o Liver
    - Advanced liver disease
  o Hemolysis
    - Hemolytic transfusion reaction
  o Blood vessels
    - Aortic aneurysm
    - Giant hemangiomas
  o Trauma
    - Massive trauma
    - Burns
  o Obstetrical disorders
    - Abruptioplacanta
    - Amniotic fluid embolism
    - Retained dead fetus

Abbreviations: DIC, disseminated intravascular coagulation.

Adapted from: Ghosh AK. *Mayo Clinic Scientific Press* 2008, page 450.

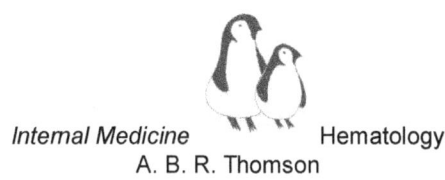

➢ Laboratory

- ○ ↑ PT
- ○ ↑ aPTT (severe DIC)
- ○ ↓ fibrinogen ⎤ intravascular coagulation
- ○ ↑ D-dimer ⎦
- ○ ↓ platelets

➢ Treatment

- ○ DIC-associated disorders
  - Obstetrical complications
  - Infection
  - Tissue injury
  - Tumours
    - Solid
    - Leukemia, acute (APL)
  - Bites spider venom
- ○ Transfusion
  - Plasma
  - Platelets
  - Cryoprecipitate

THERAPEUTIC CHALLENGE

- Give the treatment of pulmonary embolus in a patient with cirrhosis and coagulopathy.

  - ○ The coagulation abnormalities which are part of the coagulopathy of liver disease do not result in "autoanticoagulation" to the point that protects them from venous thromboembolism (↑ anticoagulation, but ↑ procoagulant production)
  - ○ Heparin followed by warfarin may be necessary.

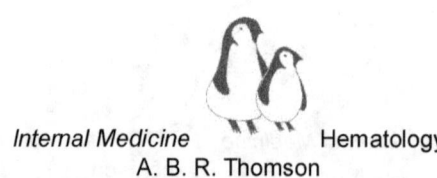

von Willebrand Disease (vWD)

➢ Definition

- o Autosomal disorder in which there is ↓ vWF (von Willebrand factor), thereby allowing more factor VIII degradation

➢ Treatment

- o Treat with desmopressin or vWF-containing factor VIII concentrates

- Give the reason why a woman who suffers from mucocutaneous bleeding and is on the oral contraceptive pill (OCP) must still be considered to have possible von Willebrand diseases even if the von Willebrand factor (vWF) is borderline low.

  - o The OCP will increase vWF, as also will exercise, stress, bleeding and inflammation.

- Give the reason why factor ~ VIIa may need to be given to the post-partum woman with bleeding and ↑aPTT, not corrected with mixing with normal plasma.

  - o An ↑aPTT, not corrected with maxing with normal plasma, suggests the presence of an acquired inhibitor to factor VIII, developing in association with pregnancy.
  - o In the setting, factor rVIIa ".... acts to bypass the need for factor VIII by binding to the surface of activated platelets, where it can generate factor Xa, leading to the production of a burst of thrombin and the formation of fibrin" (MKSAP 16, Hematology and Oncology 2012, page 168).

- A woman has severe menorrhagia, and her mother had a postpartum hemorrhage. Lab's studies show ↑aPTT but normal PT. The bleeding time and the Platelet Function Analyzer (PFA-100®) are normal. Give the likely diagnosis and recommended studies to prove the diagnosis.

  - o She likely has von Willebrand disease, in which the level of vWF may be falsely low with
    - Use of bleeding time, or Platelet Function Analyzer (PFA100®)
    - Bleeding

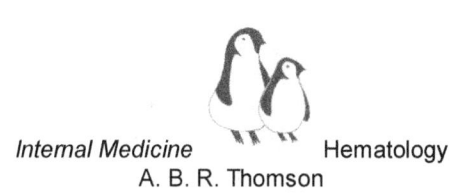

Internal Medicine   Hematology
A. B. R. Thomson

- Exercise
- Inflammation
- Stress
- Use of estrogens

➤ Pathogenesis
- o vWF (von Willebrand factor)
- o Platelets stick to injured vessels
- o Carries VIII

➤ Clinical
- o Primary and secondary failure of homeostasis due to associated ↓ VIII in vWD

➤ Diagnosis
- o PT normal
- o aPTT – N/↑
- o ↑ bleeding time
- o VIII, N/↓
- o ↓ vWF antigen
- o vWF activity assay
- o Multimer study (for vWD subtypes)

Abbreviation: vWF, von Willebrand factor

➤ Treatment
- o DDAVP (1-deamino-8-D-arginine vasopressin)
- o VIII concentrate, "intermediate purity"

Abnormal Uterine Bleeding

Interesting stats:

In adolescent women with menorrhagia, ~20% have von Willebrand disease

---

- Give the reason why vWD associated with VIII deficiency is not treated with cryoprecipitate.

  o Cryoprecipitate has a greater risk of infusion infection than does intermediate purity VIII concentrate.

TRANSFUSION MEDICINE

o 1 "unit"	- RBC
	▪ ↑ hemoglobin 1 g/dL
	- Platelets
	▪ ↑ platelets 20,000-30,000 /mL
	- Iron ~ 250 µg
o FFP	- Coagulation factors
o Cryoprecipitates	- VIII, vWF, fibrinogen

o There are many **indications** for RBC transfusions. The interested reader is referred to a general text of their choice in Internal Medicine, or reviews such as UpToDate or MKSAP 16, Hematology and Oncology 2012, Table 19, page 37.

o RBC **targets** for recipients who are actively bleeding

Coronary artery disease (CAD)	Target Hb for transfusion
No	70 g/L (7 g/dL)
Yes	100 g/L (10 g/dL)

Note: In the patient who has CAD plus possible bleeding from esophageal varices (EV), there is a fine balance for transfusion target

o Too low	- May develop cardiac ischemia
o Too high	- EV may rebleed

- For the following clinical conditions, give the lower concentration (threshold) at which platelet transfusions should be initiated.

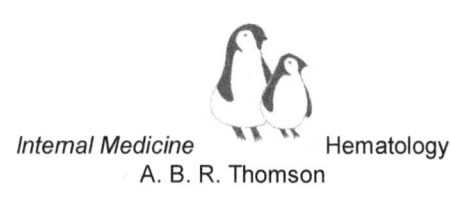

Clinic condition	Threshold for transfusion

- ➢ Thrombocytopenia, plus
    - o No risk factors — Platelets < 10,000 / μL
    - o Bleeding into lung, head (cranium) — Platelets < 40,000

- ➢ Anemia, plus
    - o Most patients — < 7.0 g/dL
    - o Acute myocardial infarction — < 10 g/dL

Adapted from Board Basics 2013, Hematology, Study Table, page 162.

- Give 3 advantages of performing pretransfusion leukoreduction.
    - o ↓ HLA alloimmunization
    - o ↓ non-hemolytic febrile reactions
    - o ↓ CMV transmission

- Give the source of preformed alloantibodies in persons receiving blood transfusions.
    - o Multiple transfused persons may receive mismatched antigens from previous transfusions
    - o Blood from multi-porous women as donors

- Give 5 methods directed at the preparation of blood for transfusion which are intended to prevent 5 types of non-hemolytic transfusion reactions.

Non-hemolytic transfusion reactions	Preparation of blood product
o Acute lung injury (TRAIL)	- Exclude multiparous women as donors
o Allergic reaction	- Washing of RBCs
o Anaphylaxis	- Washing of RBCs, or
	- IgA-deficient donors
o CMV transmission	- Leukoreduction
	- CMV-negative donor
o Febrile reaction	- Leukoreduction
o GVHD	- Irradiation of RBCs

Abbreviation: CMV, cytomegalovirus; GVHD, graft-versus-host disease; TRIAL, transfusion-related acute lung injury

Plasma Products

- o To be considered here
- o Not to be considered

- FFP (fresh frozen plasma)
- Cryoprecipitate
- α-AT
- Anti-thrombin II
- IVIG
- Protein C

Fresh Frozen Plasma (FFP)

➢ Indications
- Give 4 indications for the use of FFP transfusion.
  - o TTP
  - o DIC
  - o Liver disease
  - o Warfarin reversal (e.g. intracranial bleeding) +/- PCC
  - o Prevention of dilutional coagulation (multiple transfusion of packed RBCs)
  - o General factor replacement

➢ Dose
  - o 10 to 15 mL/kg body weight

Abbreviations: DIC, disseminated intravascular coagulation; PCC, prothrombin complex concentrate (factors II, IX and X); TTP, thromboltic thrombocytopenia purpura

Cryoprecipitate

➢ Indications
  - o Hypo-/dysfibrinogenemia
  - o Factor VIII deficiency
  - o Von Willebrand factor
  - o DIC
  - o Bleeding from thrombolytic therapy

➢ Dose
  - o 1 to 2 units per each 10 kg body weight

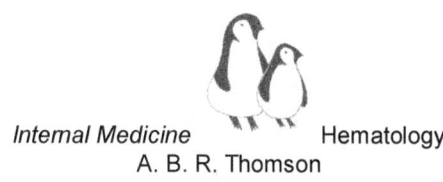

Internal Medicine   Hematology
A. B. R. Thomson

TRANSFUSION COMPLICATIONS

- Give 6 types of transfusion reactions (not infection or volume overload)

    o Acute hemolysis

    o Delayed hemolysis

    o Post-transfusion thrombocytopenia

    o Non-hemolytic febrile transfusion reaction
      - Donor WBC cytokines
      - Recipient WBC alloantibodies versus donor WBC

    o Allergic reaction

    o GVHD (graft-versus-host disease)

    o TRALI (transfusion-related acute lung injury)

To be considered here

- Give 6 major types of transfusion complications

    o Hemolytic   - Acute hemolytic transfusion reaction
                           (AHTR)
                         - Delayed hemolytic transfusion reaction
                           (DHTR)

    o No-hemolytic   - Transfusion-associated circulatory
                           overload (TACO)
                         - Transfusion-related acute lung injury
                           (TRALI)
                         - Febrile non-hemolytic transfusion
                           reaction

    o Allergic reactions and anaphylaxis

    o Transfusion associated graft-versus-host disease (T-GVHD)

    o Infection

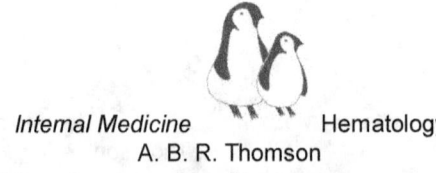

Internal Medicine　　Hematology
A. B. R. Thomson

Hemolytic Transfusion Reactions

Acute Hemolytic Transfusion Reaction (AHTR)

➤ Cause
  o ABO incompatibility between blood donor and recipient, usually arising from a clerical or technical error

➤ Clinical

    o General   - Fever
                         - Pain at infusion site

    o CVS   - Hypotension

    o Renal   - AKI (acute kidney injury)

    o Blood   - DIC

Delayed Hemolytic Transfusion Reaction

➤ Definition: ".…. an amnestic response to a performed erythrocyte alloantibody after re-exposure to an erythrocyte antigen outside the HBO system" (MKSAP 16, Hemolytic and Oncology, 2012, page 40).

➤ Clinical
  o Extravascular hemolysis ~ 1 wk after transfusion
  o DHTR in persons with sickle disease → pain crisis

Non-Hemolytic Transfusion Reactions

Transfusion-associated circulatory overload (TACO)

  o Fluid overload causing HF (heart failure) 1 to 2 hr after transfusion
  o Treatment
    - Slow infusion rate
    - Supplement O_2
    - Diuretics

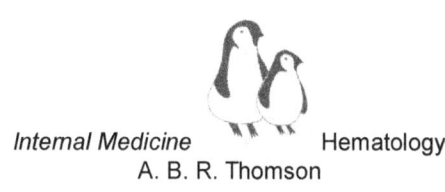

Transfusion-related Acute Lung Injury (TRALI)

➢ Definition
- o Antibodies in the plasma of the donor are directed against antigens on the neutrophils of the recipient, leading to sequestration in the lungs, damage to the capillaries, and within 6 hr of hemolysis

➢ Clinical
- o Good prognosis with supportive care
- o Donor should not provide for transfusion

Febrile Non-hemolytic Transfusion Reaction

➢ Pathogenesis
- o Cytokines from the donor plus leukoreactive antibodies from the recipient cause an early febrile reaction.

➢ Clinical
- o Stop transfusion
- o Exclude AHTR

➢ Prevention
- o Give acetaminophen
- o Continue transfusion
- o Pretransfusion antipyretics
- o Leukoreduction of future transfusion products

Allergic Reactions and Anaphylaxis

➢ Types
- o Mild   - Caused by donor plasma proteins

- o Severe   - Recipients, who are often IgA deficient, have anti-IgA antibodies which react to donor IgA

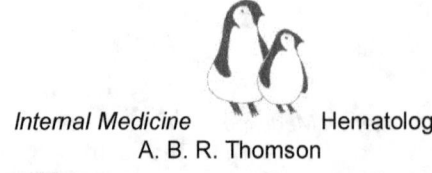

Internal Medicine   Hematology
A. B. R. Thomson

- ➢ Pathogenesis
  - ○ Donor plasma reacts with IgE on recipient's mast cells

- ➢ Treatment
  - ○ Epinephrine, IV fluids
  - ○ Stop transfusion

- ➢ Prevention
  - ○ Wash cellular products to remove plasma proteins from blood
  - ○ Use IgA-deficient donors

SO YOU WANT TO BE A HEMATOLOGIST!

A patient which thrombocytopenia is transfused 1 unit of platelets but their platelet count increases only 5000 /mL.
- Give the mechanisms for a platelet infusion to fail to ↑ platelets > 20,000 / mL.
  - ○ ↑ platelet consumption
    - fever
    - sepsis
  - ○ Antibodies developing to platelet antigens

It is widely appreciated that the blood donor who is Group O can be given to anyone, and Rh-positive can receive blood which is either Rh-positive or negative.
- Give the nature of the
  - ○ The recipient for AB plasma and platelets
    - anyone may receive AB plasma or platelets
  - ○ The blood or platelets which can be given to a Rh-negative recipient?
    - Must receive Rh-negative products

Non-hemolytic Febrile Transfusion Reaction

Pathogenesis	Prevention
○ WBC – cytokines of donor	- WBC reduction before storage
○ WBC – recipient allo-antibodies donor WBC	- WBC reduction before storage, or - WBC filtration at bedside (↓ WBC during transfusion)

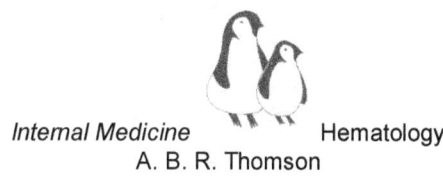

- ➢ Treatment
  - o Corticosteroids
  - o Acetaminophen / ASA

Transfusion-associated GVHD (graft-versus-host disease)

- ➢ Definition
  - o Donor lymphocytes become engrafted in an immune compromised recipient, causing damage to skin, GI mucosa, and pancytopenia

- ➢ Pathogenesis
  - o Lymphocytes of donor engraft in an immunocompromised recipient

- ➢ Persons at risk
  - o Premature infants
  - o Chemotherapy patients
  - o 1st-degree relative of donor

- ➢ Clinical
  - o Donor lymphocyte damage to
    - Skin
    - Bone marrow
    - Liver
    - GI tract

- ➢ Prevention
  - o Gamma irradiation of cellular blood components in at-risk population

- ➢ Prognosis
  - o Often fatal

- ➢ Treatment
  - o Supportive only
    - No proven effective treatment

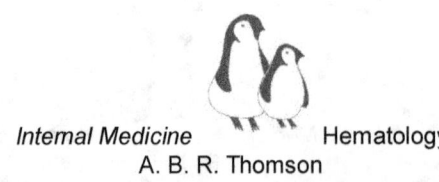

Internal Medicine   Hematology
A. B. R. Thomson

Infection

Viral infection	Risk per million (10^6)
HIV	0.5
HCV	1
HBV	< 30

- Other infections of concerns
  - WNV (West Nile virus)
  - CJD (Creutzfeldt-Jakob disease)
  - Chagas disease
  - Babesiosis

- Give the name of the bacterial organism which may cause fatal sepsis from a platelet transfusion.

  - Yersinia enterocolitica from platelets stored at room temperature

Therapeutic Apheresis

➢ Definition
  - "..... the separation of whole blood into its components, treatment or removal of the affected components, treatment or removal of the affected component, and return of the remaining blood products" (MKSAP 12, Hematology and Oncology, 2012, page 41).
  - Plasmapheresis
    - Removal of patient plasma with replacement of donor plasma (plasma exchange or an albumin / saline mixture"

CLINICAL CAUTION

Beware the development of hypocalcemia in the patient treated with therapeutic apheresis.

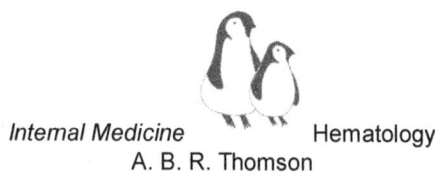

- Give 10 indications for therapeutic apheresis (standard first-line, or supportive adjuvant therapy)

System	Primary	Adjuvant
o CNS / PNS	- Acute / chronic demyelinating polyneuropathy - Myasthenia gravis - IgM-related polyneuropathy	- Lambert-Eaton syndrome - Acute CNS MS
o Blood	- Cryoglobulinemia TTP - Sickle cell disease with end-organ complications - Acute leukemia with leukocytosis	- Thrombocytosis with symptoms
o Kidney	- Good Pasteur syndrome - GP (WG)-related RPGN - Renal transplant rejection, antibody mediated	- Myeloma cast nephropathy
o Endocrine		
o Metabolic	- Familial homozygous - Hypercholesterolemia	
o Infection		- Severe malaria
o CVS		- Cardiac transplantation rejection

Abbreviations: CNS, central nervous system; GP, granulomatosis with polyangiitis; MS, multiple sclerosis; PNS, peripheral nervous system; RPGN, rapidly progressive glomerulonephritis; WG, Wegener granulomatosis

Adapted from: MKSAP 16, Hematology and Oncology, 2012, Table 21, page 41.

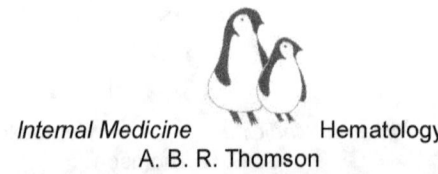

Internal Medicine   Hematology
A. B. R. Thomson

CLINICAL ALERT

In the patient with treated systemic hypertension, give the class of medications must be stopped 24 hr before elective therapeutic apheresis

---

FEBRILE NEUTROPENIA

In a patient with leukemia and antibiotic treatment who develop febrile neutropenia, suspect angioinvasive aspergillosis. If chest X-ray shows infiltration perform CT chest.

- Give the CT chest findings in the patient with invasive aspergillosis.

    - o Infiltrates
        - Nodular
        - Patchy
        - Ground-glass "halo" sign

- ➤ Treatment
    - o Start with anti-pseudomonas
        - Meropenem
        - Imipenem
        - Cefepime
        - Pip-tazo (piperacillin-tazobactam)

    - o If poor response, add
        - Aminoglycoside
        - Fluoroquinolone +/-
        - Vancomycin

    - o Do <u>not</u> use
        - Colony-stimulating factors for neutropenia
        - Anti-viral therapy, unless there is evidence for a viral infection

PLASMA CELL DYSCRASIAS

- ➤ Definition
    - o "... abnormal clonal proliferation of immunoglobulin-secreting differentiated B-lymphoid cells and plasma cells.
    - o A malignancy of plasma cells involving bone and bone marrow (≥ 10% clonal plasma cells), with

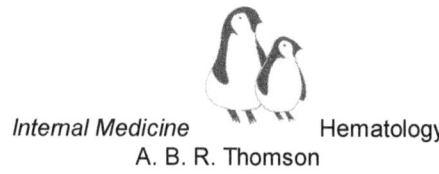

Internal Medicine Hematology
A. B. R. Thomson

o ↑ production of M (monoclonal) protein (≥ 3 g / dL)
  - ↑ heavy chain   IgG, IgA or IgD, +/-
  - ↑ light chain   κ, λ
  - Non-secretory disease is rare
o End-organ damage

Source: Board Basics 2013, Hematology, page 163.

➤ Types
- o Multiple myeloma
- o MGUS (monoclonal gammopathy of undetermined significance)
- o Waldenström's macroglobulinemia
- o AL amyloidosis (light-chain-associated amyloidosis)

➤ Clinical
- o Bone
  - Vertebral compression fractures
  - Osteopenia / osteoporosis
  - Lytic bone lesions
  - Hypercalcemia
- o Blood anemia
- o Kidney disease

o Bone pain from lytic lesions

o Spinal cord compression

o Blood
  - Anemia
  - Leukopenia
  - Thrombocytopenia

o Lab: ↑ serum
  - Creatinine
  - Calcium
  - M protein (97%)

• Give 4 common renal abnormalities in multiple myeloma.

o ↑ serum creatinine

o Cast nephropathy

o AL amyloidosis

o Albuminuria

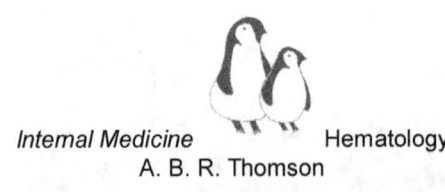

Internal Medicine   Hematology
A. B. R. Thomson

- o M protein
- o Treatment related
  - FSG (focal segmental glomerulosclerosis) from pamidronate for prevention of pathological fractures
  - ATN (acute tubular necrosis) from zoledronic acid (bisphosphonate)

CLINICAL ALERT

About half of patients with multiple myeloma have renal injury, which can be worsened by nephrotoxic drugs such as NSAIDs

---

➢ Diagnosis
- o Serum, urine
  - ↑ monoclonal M protein
- o Bone marrow
  - ↑ clonal plasma cells,
  - Plasmacytoma
- o MGUS
  - ↑ Serum monoclonal protein, but < 3 gm
  - Bone marrow ↑ clonal plasma cells, but < 10%
  - No end-organ damage in bone, blood, kidney
- o AL amyloidosis
  - Serum / urine light-chains
  - May also affect tongue, liver, heart

➢ Spectrum: important factors
- o M protein serum
- o % bone marrow plasma cells
- o B2 microglobulin (serum)
- o End-stage damage
  - Serum Ca^{2+} > 2.6 mmol/L (> 10.5 mg/dL)
  - Serum creatinine > 1777 µmol/L (> 2 mg/dL)
  - Hemoglobin
    - < 100 g/L (< 10 g/dL), or
    - 20 g/L < LLN (2 g/dL < LLN)

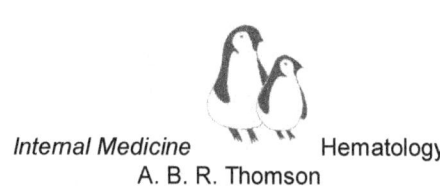

- Bone disease
- Hyperviscosity syndrome
- AL amyloidosis
- Recurrent bacterial infections

Diagnosis of dyscrasis	M protein > 3 g/dL	Bone marrow plasma cells ≥ 10, %	MROD	S B2-microglobulin
MGUS	-	-	-	-
↓ 1% per yr				
Myeloma Asymptomatic*	+	+	-	-
↓				
Symptomatic	+	+	+	Stage I* > 3.5 mg/L II in between III > 5.5 mg/L

*May have M protein ≥ 3 g/dL and/or ≥ 10% bone marrow plasma cells
* in stage I, serum albumin ≥ 35 g/L (3.5 g/dL)

Abbreviations: MGUS, monoclonal gammopathy of undetermined significance

- Give 3 risk factors for the progression of asymptomatic to symptomatic MM (multiple myeloma)

  o M protein concentration

  o % of plasma cells in bone marrow

  o ↑ free light chains ⎤
  ⎬ ↓ serum K⁺ / free light chains
  o ↓ non-clonal light chains ⎦

➢ Treatment
  o Pharmaceutical
    - Melphalan
      ▪ Alkylating agent
    - Corticosteroids

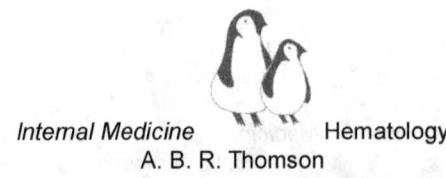

- Thalidomide, or Lenalidomide
  - Immunomodulatory
- Bortezomib
  - Protease inhibitor

  o HSCT (hematopoietic stem cell transplantation)

  - Induction
    - Dexamethasone, bortezomib +/-
    - Thalidomine or lenalidomide
  - Consolidation
    - Melphalan
  - Relapses

    Bortezomib or lenalidomide

> Therapy (of multiple myeloma)
  o Indication
    - Symptoms
  o < 75 yr
    - HSCT (human stem cell transplantation)
    - Vigorous pretransplant induction chemotherapy
      - Dexamethasone plus lenalidomide or thalidomide, or
      - Bortezomib, used alone for induction or relapse
  o > 75 yr
    - Prednisone plus melphalan (do <u>not</u> use for HSCT induction therapy)
  o Care of complications
    - Bone
      - Spinal cord compression
        - Corticosteroids
        - Radiation
      - Pathological fractures
      - Osteoporosis
    - Blood
      - Hyperviscosity syndrome
        - Plasmapheresis
      - Anemia
        - Erythropoietin
    - Infections / Immunization
      - Pneumococcus
      - Influenza
      - Immunoglobulin (for frequent bacterial infections)
      - Varicella-zoster vaccine (if patient to use rescue bortezomib)

- In the context of the patient with multiple myeloma, give the symptoms which would suggest the hyperviscosity syndrome, and the need for plasmapheresis.

    o Eyes   -   Blurred vision

    o CNS   -   Altered mentation
                    -   Headaches
                    -   Fatigue

    o Heart   -   HF (heart failure)

    o GI   -   Mucosal bleeding

MELANOMA

➤ The common risk factors

    o Sunshine, especially
        - In childhood
        - Fair skin
        - Repeated sunburns

    o Cutaneous nevi

    o Family history

    o BRAF gene V600E mutation

➤ Treatment

    o Surgical excision   -   < 1 mm
                           -   No ulceration
                           -   Low intake index

    o SLNB (sentinel   -   Positive-regional lymph node dissection
      lymph node biopsy)

    o Follow-up annual
      skin examinations

    o Metastatic disease   -   IV dacarbazine
                           -   po temozolomide
                           -   Ipilimumab
                           -   Verurafenib (for patients who have
                               BRAF gene V600E mutation)

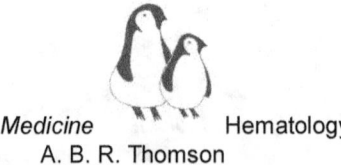

- Give the reason why melphalan is used for non-HSCT treatment of MM, and for consolidation therapy for human stem cell transplantation (HSCT), but not for induction.

  - Melphalan is toxic to stem cells, so is not used initially after HSCT.
  - Complications
    - Lytic bone disease
      - Kyphoplasty, for spinal stability
      - Radiation, for palliation of pain
      - Bisphosphonates, for prevention of pathological fractures
    - Renal failure
      - Treat ↑ serum Ca^{2+}
      - Avoid nephrotoxins
      - Plasmapheresis
    - Cast nephropathy
    - Free light chains
      Chemotherapy, for ↑ light chains

- Give the risk of treating multiple myeloma (MM) with high dose dexamethasone plus lenalidomide.

  - High risk of VTE (venous thromboembolism), approximately 8% to 16% for relapsing MM, even higher for new diagnosis of MM.

- Give the differences between multiple myeloma, and multiple myeloma syndromes.

  - Multiple myeloma
    - ≥ 10% clonal plasma cells on bone marrow biopsy
  - Multiple myeloma syndrome
    - Multiple myeloma **plus** end-organ damage

MYELOPROLIFERATIVE DISORDERS

➤ Definition: :.... a group of clonal cell disorders characterized by absent regulation of proliferation that results in excess production of myeloid elements in the bone marrow"

Source: Board Basics 2013, Hematology, page 164

➤ Types   o WBC   -   CML (chronic myeloid leukemia)

                  o Platelets   -   Essential thrombocythemia

                  o RBC   -   Polycythemia vera

                  o Fibroblasts   -   Myelofibrosis

Chronic Myeloid Leukemia (CML)

➤ Definition: "...... a hematopoietic stem cell disorder characterized by myeloid proliferation associated with a (9; 22) (q 34: q 11) translocation, the Philadelphia chromosome.

➤ Clinical
     o CML may undergo
         - Accelerated phase (blasts cells are 10%-20% of leucocytes)
         - Blast crisis (blast cells are > 20% of leucocytes)

     o Transformation into
         - Acute leukemia
             ▪ Myeloid
             ▪ Lymphoid

➤ Diagnosis
     o Cytogenic study of bone marrow – Philadelphia chromosome
     o Bcr-abl gene

➤ Treatment
     o Often no treatment required
     o Young, accelerated phase / blast crisis
         - HSCT

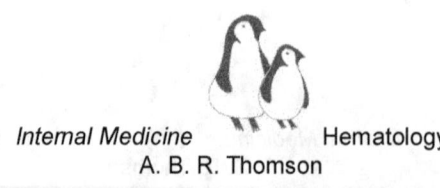

- o Disease control / molecular remission
  - Imatinib mesylate
  - Dasatinib
  - Nilotinib
- o Palliation hydroxyurea
- o Platelet transfusion
  - Bleeding < 10,000 /mL
- o Splenectomy
  - Painful splenomegaly
  - Multiple transfusion requirements
  - Despite imatinib mesylate or hydroxyurea

Conventional cytogenic testing may miss subtle changes which would elute the diagnosis of CML (chronic myeloid leukemia).

- Give the value of FISH (fluorescence in situ hybridization) to diagnose CML.

  - o FISH testing of the peripheral blood is sensitive to detect (9;22) translocations

- Give the limitation of flow cytometry of peripheral blood to diagnose CML.

  - o Flow cytometry is limited in its role to diagnose CML because the CML cells
    - Are not varying stages of myelopoiesis
    - Do not express aberrant cell surface

Essential Thrombocythemia

- ➤ Definition
  - o Platelet count > 600 x 10⁹ /L (600,000 µL) on 2 different accasions separated by at least 1 month in a person with no other cause for thrombocythemia
  - o Pathogenesis of bleeding disorder

- o Myeloproliferative disorder-characterized by
  - Platelets > 600,000 mL
  - ↑ Bone marrow megakaryocytes
  - Clinical complications of
    - Thrombosis
    - Hemorrhage
  - Associated with JAK2 mutation (in 50%)

➢ Mechanism

• Give the mechanism of the bleeding disorder in essential thrombocythemia.

- o ↑↑ platelets   - Qualitative dysfunction similar to vWD (von Willebrand disease)

➢ Clinical

- o ~ ½ have mutation in JAK2
- o Hepatomegaly, ~20%

  - o CNS
    - Headaches
    - Visual disturbance
    - TIA / CVA

  - o Skin
    - Erythromelalgia (red, warm, swollen, painful hands or feet)
    - Livedo reticularis

  - o Splenomegaly (in 50%)

  - o CVS
    - CAD (coronary obstruction / ischemia) / MI (myocardial infarction)

  - o GI
    - Bleeding

➢ Laboratory
  - o Peripheral blood
    - Megakaryocytes
    - Leucocytosis
    - Basophilia
  - o Bone marrow
    - Hypercellular
    - Hyperplasia of megakaryocytes
    - Clusters of megakaryocytes

Internal Medicine   Hematology
A. B. R. Thomson

➢ Treatment

o	No symptoms	- ASA 81 mg po OD Follow-up
o	Erythromelalgia	- ASA 81 mg po OD
o	Mild symptoms	- ASA 81 mg po OD, plus - Hydroxyurea, anagrelide, or IFN (interferon alpha)
o	Severe	- CNS, CVS, GI symptoms: Hydroxyurea plus platelet apheresis

Polycythemia vera (PV)

➢ Clinical (thrombosis and bleeding)

- o ↑↑↑ RBC mass ↑ hematocrit
  - M > 60%
  - W > 56%
- o ↑ WBC and platelet
- o JAK2 V617F mutation (in 95%)
- o ↓ erythropoietin
- o Splenomegaly
- o ↑ cellularity in bone marrow

➢ Clinical

o	CNS	- Headaches - TIA / CVA
o	CVS	- MI - DVT
o	GI	- BCS (Budd-Chiari syndrome)
o	Skin	- Facial plethora - Erythromelalgia - ↑ pruritis with hot water

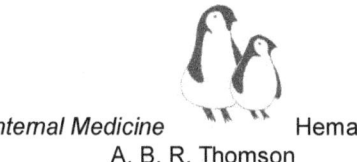

➢ Therapy
- o Phlebotomy
  - Lower hematocrit
    - M > 60% → < 45%
    - F > 56% → < 42%
- o Hydroxyurea
  - \> 60 yr
  - Previous thrombosis
- o ASA 81 mg po OD
- o Allopurinol for hyperuricemia
- o Anti-histamines
  - Pruritis

- Give the reason why low-dose rather than standard-/high dose ASA is given for PV (polycythemia vera) or for ET (essential thrombocythemia).

  - o PV and ET are associated with thrombosis and bleeding
  - o Low-dose ASA will ↓ risk of thrombosis, but high-dose ASA would ↑ risk of bleeding (while ↓ risk of thrombosis)

- Give the diagnostic features of polycythemia vera.

  - o Hb (hemoglobin concentration, g/L [g/dL] >
    - Women 165 (16.5)
    - Men 185 (18.5)

  - o Leucytosis

  - o Thrombocytosis

  - o Hepatosplenomegaly

  - o Mutation JAK1 VG17F

BUZZ WORDS

- o Itchy skin after a bath (!)
- o Philadelhia chromosome (BCR-ABL)
- o Craving for ice cubes (!)
- o ↑aPTT failing to correct with normal plasma ("mixing test"

- Polycythemia vera
- CML (chronic myeloid leukemia)
- Iron deficiency (!)
- Acquired hemophilia (acquired antibody to factor VIII)

- Give the role of measuring blood erythropoietin concentration in the patient with polycythemia (erythrocytosis).

Type of polycythemia	Erythropoietin lever
Primary	↓
Secondary	↑

Myelofibrosis with Myeloid Metaplasia (MMM)

➤ Pathogenesis

- o Clonal proliferation of abnormal hematopoietic stem cells in the bone marrow release cytokines which ↑ production of fibroblasts

- o ↑ fibroblasts fibrosis of marrow, and marrow failure

SO YOU WANT TO BE A HEMATOLOGIST!

- Give a description of the peripheral blood smear of the patient with myelofibrosis with myeloid metaplasia.

    - o RBC
        - Tear drop
        - Nucleated
        - Erythroblasts

    - o Platelets
        - Giant

➤ Clinical
- o Bone marrow failure → extramedullary hematopoiesis → splenomegaly / hepatomegaly → PHT (portal hypertension)
- o MMM may transform into acute leukemia
- o < 60 yr
    - HSCT
- o > 60 yr
    - Supportive therapy

Bony Sclerosis

Sclerotic lesions may be seen in the skull of persons with myelofibrosis

- Give a systematic approach to the causes of sclerosis (increase in bone density).

  o Long bones
    - Paget disease
    - Metastases
      - Prostate
      - Breast
      - Reticuloses
      - Usually in spine, pelvis,ribs
      - May grow outside the confines of the bone, unlike Paget disease
    - Chronic osteomyelitis
    - Myelofibrosis
    - Avascular necrosis
    - Marble bone disease (osteopetrosis)
    - Fluorosis

  o Skull
    - Meningioma hyperostosis frontalis

Adapted from: Davies IJT. *Lloyd-Luke (medical books) LTD* 1972, page 221.

Trick and Red Herings

- Give the reasons why splenectomy is not performed in MMM (myelofibrosis with myeloid metaplasia)

  o No survival benefit
  o ↑ risk of
    - Transformation of MMM to leukemia
    - Hemorrhage
    - Thrombosis

CHRONIC MYELOID DISORDERS

Myelodysplastic Syndromes (MDS)

➢ Presentation
  o Refractory anemia plus, ↑ blasts-2
  o Unilineage (or multi-lineage) dysplasia

➢ Cause
  o Malignant clonal abnormalities usually affecting chromosomes 3, 5, 7, 8 and 17
  o These clonal abnormalities result in
    - Cytopenia in ≥ 2 of 3 call lines (RBC
      ↑ MCV
      Nucleated
      Teardrop

➢ Clinical course
  o Worsening anemia leucopenia, thrombocytopenic
  o Transformation to acute leukemia
  o Bone marrow failure

➢ Differential
  o Deficiency of folate / cobalamin
    - Alcohol
    - Drugs
    - Myeloproliferative disorders

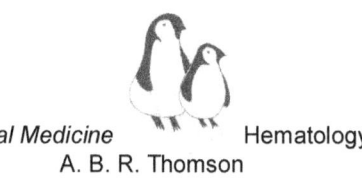

➤ Therapy   o Asymptomatic   -   Follow-up

                          o Symptoms   -   Erythropoietin
- GCSF (granulocyte colony-stimulating factor)
- HSCT

                          o 5q subgroup of   -   Lenalidomide
                              MDS

- A higher risk myelodysplastic syndrome (MDS) is diagnosed. Give the recommended therapy for newly diagnosed MDS.

  o Azacitidine

SO YOU WANT TO BE A HEMATOLOGIST!

- Give the difference between "myeloid metaplasia" and "extramedullary hematopoiesis"?

  o None: they both represent ectopic hematopoietic activity, usually in liver and spleen, and may not be associated with myelofibrosis (bone marrow fibrosis).

- Give the meaning of "myelofibrosis with myeloid metaplasia"?

  o By convention, is idiopathic myelofibrosis

Hematopoietic Growth Factors

Indications for use

  o ESAs (erythrocyte-stimulating agents [epopetin, darbepoetin alfa])
  - Cancer-related symptomatic anemia (hemoglobin ≤ 100 g/L [≤ 10 g / dL) when chemotherapy is not curative
  - Chronic renal failure +/- hemodialysis when hemoglobin < 100 g / L
  - Serum iron saturation should be ≥ 20%, and serum failure 100 – 200 μg / mL (100 – 200 ng / mL)

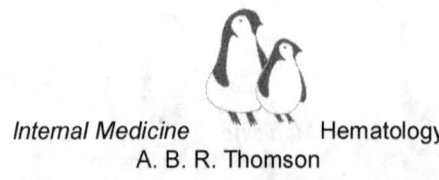

- o G-CSF and GM-CSF (granulocyte-macropahge colony-stimulating factor)
    - Primary prophylaxis for neutropenia in persons undergoing myelosuppression
    - Persons with non-malignant disease who have infection associated with neutropenia

- o Thrombopoietin
    - Relapsing ITP (idiopathic thrombocytopenic purpura)

Chemotherapy-Induced Myelodysplastic Syndrome

➢ Definition
- o Myelodysplastic syndromes are stem cell disorders which cause hypercellular bone marrow dyserythropoiesis, which in turn causes ineffective hematopoiesis and peripheral cytopenias, with onset months to years after chemo- or radiotherapy

➢ Diagnosis
- o Bone marrow cytogenetic studies show chromosomal changes, without lymphadenopathy or hepatosplenomegaly

EPSTEIN-BARR VIRUS (EBV) INFECTION

➢ Clinical

Although EBV infection is usually associated with infectious mononucleosis syndrome (IMS) (flu-like illness, fever, posterior cervical lymphoadenopathy, aplenomegaly, sore throat, measles-like rash after ampicillin, atypical peripheral blood lymphocytes and positive serology), some patients may have atypical presentations.

- Give 4 presentations of EBV infection other than the typical IMS or EBV-associated malignancies.

    - o CNS   - Aseptic meningitis
                   - Aseptic encephalitis

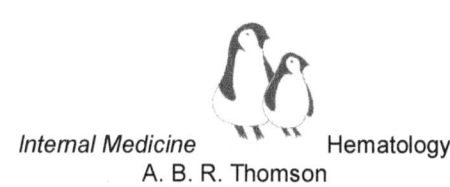

- o Liver   -   Hepatitis
- o Blood   -   Hemolytic anemia
  -   Thrombocytopenia

- Give 3 viruses which are associated with IMS (infectious mononucleosis syndrome)

  - o EBV
  - o CMV
  - o HIV

➢ Complications

- Give 4 malignant or premalignant conditions associated with EBV

  - o Lymphoma   -   B-cell lymphoma
    -   T-cell lymphoma
    -   Hodgkin lymphoma
    -   PTLD (post-transplantation lymphoproliferative disorder)

  - o Leukoplakia,   -   Painless, white, corrugated plaques on edge of
    Or   tongue

  - o Nasopharyngeal carcinoma

  - o   Hodgkin lymphoma may be due to EBV (Ebstein Barr Virus)
  - o An entire lymph node must be examined histologically to distinguish from non-Hodgkin lymphoma, such as
    -   Burkitt lymphoma
    -   Diffuse large B-cell lymphoma

Beware the "company" that diseases keep.

In the patient with oral hairy leukoplakia, in addition to EBV infection, give the other viral infection which must be excluded.

    Oral hairy leukoplakia is highly suggestive of an infection with HIV

➤ Diagnosis

• Give the serological tests for present and past EBV infection.

	EBV Infection	
	Present acute primary	Past
○ Viral capsid antigen IgM	↑	0
○ Early antigen IgE	↑	0
○ Epstein-Barr nuclear antigen-1 IgE	↓ / 0	↑

Note; VCA (viral capsid antigen) IgG is increased in both, thus does not help to distinguish between present and past EBV infection

➤ Treatment

   ○ Conservative

   ○ No anti-viral drugs

   ○ Corticosteroids for severe
      - Lung disease
      - Hemolytic anemia

LYMPHADENOPATHY AND MASS IN HEAD, NECK AND AXILLA

For a list of the common sites and characteristics of lymphadenopathy, please see: Filate W, et al. Essentials of Clinical Examination Handbook. 5th Edition. *The Medical Society, Faculty of Medicine, University of Toronto*, 2005, pages 120 and 121.

➤ Clinical: Generalized Lymph Node Enlargement
   ○ Examine the mouth for the following signs:
      - Tonsillar lymph nodes
      - Palatal petechiae and pharyngitis (glandular fever)
      - Neoplastic tumors and ulcers

   ○ Examine other lymph node areas in a systemic manner: submental, submadibular, deep cervical (upper and lower), occipital, posterior triangle, supraclavicular, axillary, epitrochlear and inguinal

   ○ Upper cervical lymph nodes: examine the chest, breast and upper limbs. Also, perform an ear, nose and throat (ENT) examination for nasopharyngeal carcinoma

   ○ Lower cervical and supraclavicular lymph nodes: examine the thyroid, chest, abdomen for gastric carcinoma (Virchow's nodes) and testis

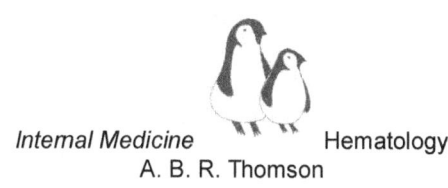

    o Axillary lymph nodes: examine the chest, breast and upper limbs

    o Inguinal lymph nodes: examine the lower limbs and external genitalia

For the differential diagnosis of neck mass, please see: Filate W, et al. Essentials of Clinical Examination Handbook. 5th Edition. *The Medical Society, Faculty of Medicine, University of Toronto*, 2005, page 106.

- Give the performance characteristics for lymphadenopathy.

Finding	PLR	NLR
➢ General		
o Age ≥ 40 years	2.4	0.4
o Weight loss	3.4	0.8
➢ Distribution of Adenopathy		
o Supraclavicular nodes	3.2	0.8
➢ Characteristics of Adenopathy		
o Lymph node size		
– ≥ 9 cm^2	8.4	
o Hard texture	3.2	0.6
o Fixed lymph nodes	10.9	NS
➢ Lymph Node Score		
5 or 6	5.1	
7 or more	21.9	

Abbreviation: NLR, negative likelihood ratio; PLR, positive likelihood ration. Note that there a number of findings which are not listed here, because their PLR is < 2. These include male sex, fever, head and neck nodes (excluding supraclavicular nodes), axillary nodes, inguinal nodes, epitrochear nodes, generalized lymphadenopathy, lymph node size < 4 cm or 4 - 8.99 cm^2, lymph node tenderness, rash, palpable spleen, palpable liver, lymph node score ≤ 4.

Probability

        Decrease   Increase

-45%	-30%	-15%		+15%	+30%	+45%	
0.1	0.2	0.5	1	2	5	10	LRs

Adapted from: McGee SR. *Saunders/Elsevier* 2007, Box 24.1, page 292.

Clinical pearl: *90% of pediatric neck masses are inflammatory, whereas 90% of adult neck masses are metastatic.*

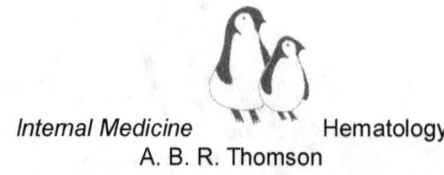

Internal Medicine   Hematology
A. B. R. Thomson

> Lymph nodes of head, neck and axilla

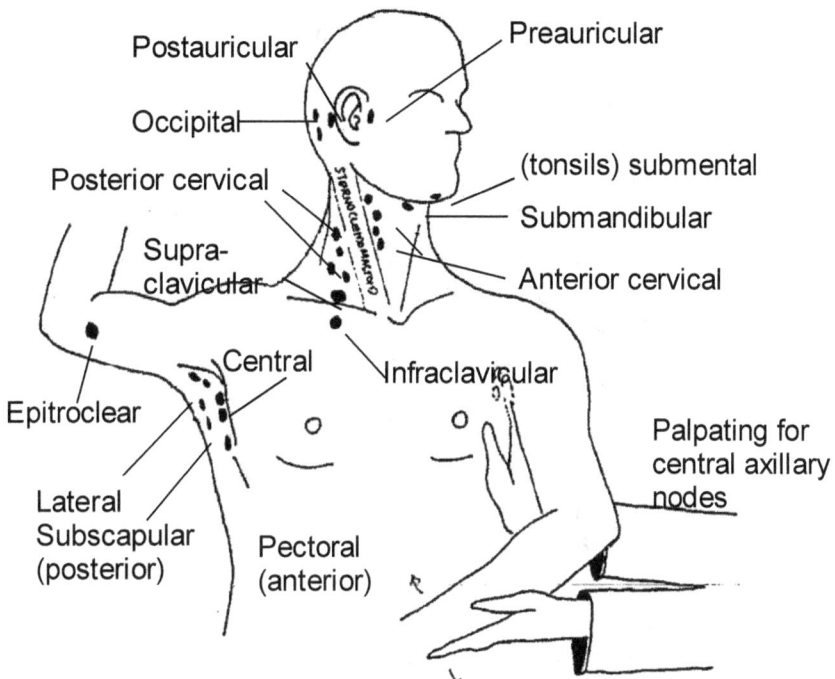

Reproduced with the permission of Dr. B. Fisher, University of Alberta

Useful background: Perform a focused examination for cervical lymphadenopathy

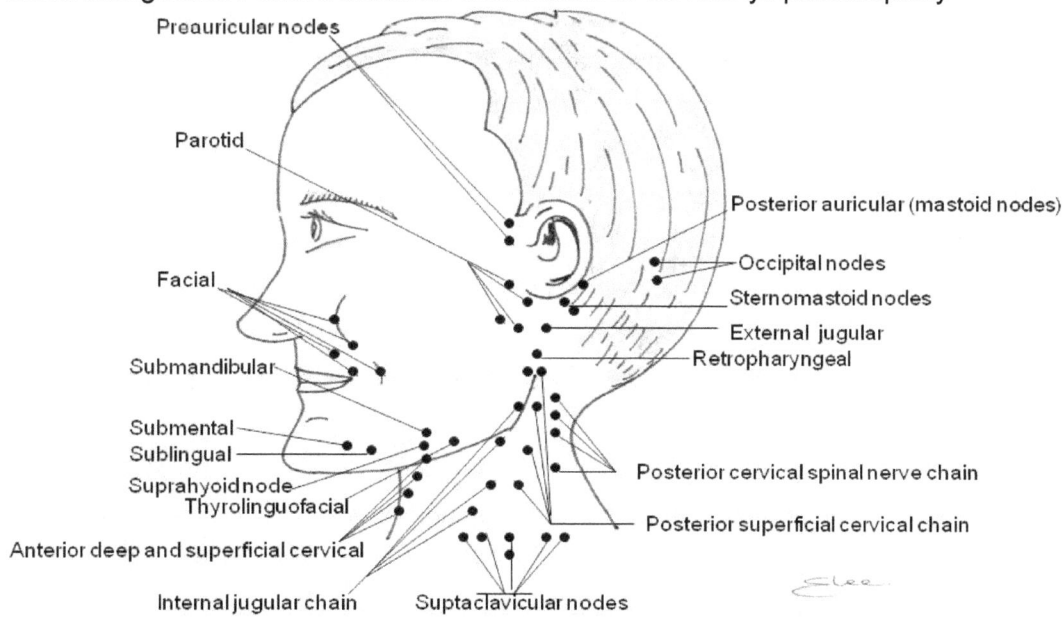

Adapted from: Mangione S. *Hanley & Belfus* 2000, page 401

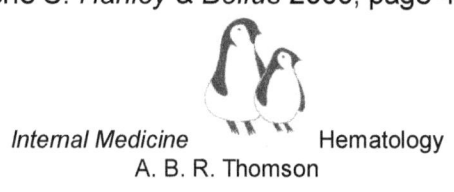

Internal Medicine   Hematology
A. B. R. Thomson

SO YOU WANT TO BE A HEMATOLOGIST!

- Give the types and causes of regional lymphadenopathy.

  - ➢ Cervical lymphadenopathy
    - o Infectious
      - Bacterial pharyngitis
      - Dental abscess
      - Otitis media
      - Infectious mononucleosis
      - Cytomegalovirus
      - Gonococcal pharyngitis
      - Toxoplasmosis
      - Hepatitis
      - Adenovirus
    - o Malignancies
      - Non-Hodgkin's disease
      - Hodgkin's disease
      - Squamous cell carcinoma of head & neck

  - ➢ Virchow node (anterior left supraclavicular lymph node). (Also known asTroiser's ganglion)
    - o Carcinoma of breast, bronchus, lymphomas and gastrointestinal neoplasms

  - ➢ Delphian node (a midline prelaryngeal lymph node)
    - o Laryngeal malignancy
    - o Heralds thyroid disease
    - o Lymphoma

  - ➢ Axillary lymphadenopathy
    - o Infectious
      - Staphylococcal
      - Streptococcal infections of the arm
      - Cat scatch fever
      - Tularaemia
      - Sporotrichosis
    - o Malignant
      - Hodgkin's disease
      - Non-Hodgkin's lymphoma
      - Carcinoma of breast and melanoma

  - ➢ Epitrochlear lymphadenopathy
    - o Most common causes are lymphoma/CLL and infectious mononucleosis
    - o Other diagnoses include HIV, sarcoidosis, and connective tissue disorders
    - o In developing countries secondary syphilis, lepromatous leprosy, leishmaniasis and rubella are important causes.

Printed with permission: Baliga RR. *Saunders/Elsevier* 2007, pages 570 and 571.

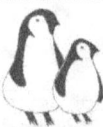

Internal Medicine   Hematology
A. B. R. Thomson

- Give the lymph node area, source of drainage, and causes of common lymphadenopathy

Lymph node area	Area of drainage

➢ Head and neck

 o Pre-/ postauricular — Eye, scalp

 o Occipital — Posterior scalp

 o Submental — Lower face, floor of mouth

 o Submandibular — Face, oral cavity

 o Cervical
  - Anterior   Pharynx, tonsils, face, scalp
  - Posterior   Posterior scalp, ear

➢ Clavicular/ axillary

 o Clavicular
  - Supra-/ infraclavicular   Cervical lymph node chains, abdomen, thorax, arm and breast

 o Axillary   Other axillary nodes
  - Central
  - Lateral — Most of arm
  - Posterior (subscapular) — Posterior chest wall, upper arm
  - Anterior (pectoral) — Anterior chest wall, most of breast

➢ Upper Extremities

 o Superior to the clavicle — Head, neck & axillary nodes

 o Posterior to the clavicle — Head, neck & axillary nodes

 o At apex of axilla — All other axillary nodes

 o High in axilla, deep to pectoralis minor — Pectoral, subscapular and lateral nodes

 o Along lower border of pectoralis major, inside anterior axillary fold — Anterior chest wall, most of breast

 o Along lateral border of scapula, deep in posterior axillary fold — Anterior chest wall, most of breast

 o Upper humerus — Most of arm

 o Epitrochlear (cubita) — Lower arm

 o Above medial epicondyle — Ulnar side of hand & forearm

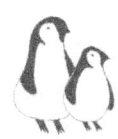

Lymph node area	Area of drainage

> Lower extremities

  o Upper portion of leg   - Superficial tissue of upper portion of leg

  o Below inguinal ligament   - Skin of
                   ▪ lower abdominal wall
                   ▪ external genitalia (not testes)
                   ▪ lower 1/3 of vagina
                   ▪ gluteal area

  o Medial aspect of femoral vein   - Popliteal node and superficial inguinal nodes

  o Popliteal fossa   - Heel and outer aspect of foot
  o Epitrochlear

Adapted from: Filate W, et al. *The Medical Society, Faculty of Medicine, University of Toronto*, 2005, pages 116-120; and Baliga RR. *Saunders/Elsevier* 2007, page 570; McGee SR. *Saunders/Elsevier* 2007, pages 116 and 117.

Neck and Axillary Lymphadenopathy

> Clinical

• Take a directed history and perform a focused physical examination for mass/lymph nodes in the neck/axilla

  o General considerations
    - Lymph nodes found in normal persons are small, mobile discrete, non-tender
    - Enlargement of a supraclavicular node suggests possible metastasis from a thoracic or an abdominal malignancy, especially on the left supraclavicular node
    - Tender nodes suggest inflammation, hard or fixed nodes suggest malignancy
    - Lymph nodes should be movable in two directions; up and down, and side-to-side (Neither a muscle nor an artery).

  o Description
    - Location and local./generalized
    - Size

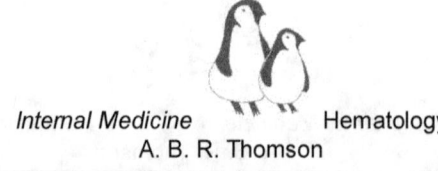

- Shape
- Consistency (hardness of node is neither sensitive nor specific of malignancy)
- Tenderness
- Mobility
- Confluence/matting with other nodes
- Dimpling or drainage to overlying skin

o Use the pneumonic **ALL AGES** to approach a patient with lymphadenopathy

o **A**ge at presentation (e.g. infectious mononucleosis is commoner in younger age groups; Hodgkin's disease has a bimodal peak).

o **L**ocation(s) of lymph nodes (lymph nodes present outside the inguinal regions, for longer than one month and measuring 1 cm x 1 cm or larger without an obvious diagnosis should be considered for biopsy)

o **L**ength of time the lymph nodes are present

o **A**ssociated symptoms and signs including fever ('B' symptoms: temp >38°C, drenching night sweats, unexplained weight loss >10% body weight)

o **G**eneralized lymph node enlargement

o **E**xtranodal organ involvement

o **S**plenomegaly (rare in metastatic cancer; consider infectious mononucleosis lymphoma, chronic lymphocytic leukemia, and acute leukemia)

Source: McGee SR. *Saunders/Elsevier* 2007, page 569.

➢ History
  o Onset of symptoms, duration, alleviating or aggravating factors, other associated symptoms, progression of symptoms
  o Unilateral/bilateral
  o Delimitation (borders)
  o Epistaxis/nasal obstruction
  o Oral pain
  o Otalgia (referred)
  o Dysphagia,hoarseness, stridor
  o Environmental/occupational exposures (e.g. radiation, asbestos)
  o Travel history
  o HIV, EBV, TB
  o Symptoms of thyroid dysfunction
  o Medications (e.g. phenytoin, allopurinol)

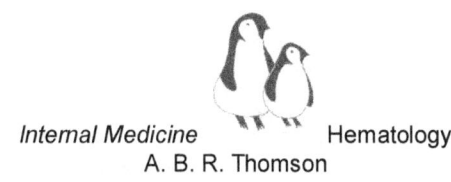

Internal Medicine   Hematology
A. B. R. Thomson

- o Exposure to animals
- o History of cancer
- o IV drug use
- o Cardiac problems, review of systems

➢ Physical examination

- Perform a directed physical examination for lymph nodes in the neck and axilla.
  - o Occipital lymph nodes
    - Located at the junction between head and neck, common in childhood infections
    - In adults, a sign of scalp infection
    - In the absence of infection, they usually reflect a generalized lymphadenopathy, such as may be encountered in HIV infection
  - o Posterior cervical lymphadenopathy
    - Dandruff or nasopharyngeal tumor
  - o Preauricular nodes
    - Lymphoma or on the same side of conjunctivitis (often referred to as Parinarud's syndrome)
  - o Nodes scattered around the two branches of the mandible
    - Localized pathology, such as periodontitis or other teeth infection
    - Or submental and submandibular nodes reflect cancer of the nose, lip, anterior tongue, or anterior floor of the mouth
  - o Midjugular nodes
    - Cancer of the base of the tongue or larynx
  - o Lower jugular nodes
    - Primary cancer of the thyroid or cervical esophagus
  - o Non-nodal findings
    - Myositis, torticollis
    - Salivary gland
      - ▪ Calculi
      - ▪ Thyroid, thyroglossal duct cyst*, thyroid tumor, goitre, or pyramidal lobe

Adapted from: Mangione S. *Hanley & Belfus* 2000, pages 400-1; Talley NJ, et al. *Maclennan & Petty Pty Limited*, 2003, page 233, 235; McGee SR. *Saunders/Elsevier*, 2007, pages 284-90; Filate W, et al. *The Medical Society, Faculty of Medicine, University of Toronto* 2005, page 119-21; and Davey P. *Wiley-Blackwell* 2006, pages 82 and 83 and Baliga RR. *Saunders/Elsevier* 2007, pages 570 -1.

ANEMIA

➤ Clinical

• Take a directed history for anemia.

• History

     o Fatigue
       - Duration
       - Onset
       - Course
       - Frequency
       - Limitations in activities

     o Associated symptoms
       - Malaise
       - Weakness
       - Dyspnea
       - Chest pain
       - Palpitations
       - Headache
       - Tinnitus
       - Presyncope/syncope
       - Craving for ice

     o Potential sites of blood loss
       - Previous past anemia
       - Menstrual bleeding (changes in frequency, amount, duration of menses)
       - Respiratory. tract hemoptysis,_epistaxis
       - GI bleeding melena, hematochezia, hematemesis
       - Urinary/ renal bleeding (hematuria)
       - Previous multiple blood donations (frequency, last donation, amount donated)

     o Dietary history
       - Iron deficiency
       - Folic acid/B12 deficiency
       - Alcohol
       - Vegans

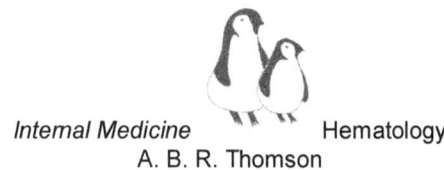

- o Past medical history
  - Chronic inflammatory disorders
  - Liver or renal disease
  - Endocrine disorders (hypo/hyperthyroid, Addison's disease)
  - Malignancies (myeloma, leukemia)
  - Alcohol use (quantity, duration)
  - Lead exposure
  - Medications (ASA, NSAIDs, chemotherapeutic agents)

- o Family medical history
  - Genetic background (Mediterranean/ African/ Asian)
  - Hereditary anemia (sideroblastosis, spherocytosis, elliptocytosis, stomatocytosis)

- Perform a focused physical examination for anemia.

o Eyes	- Palor
o Mouth	- Glossitis
o Thyroid	- Goiter
o Hands	- Palor
	- Lose of palmar crease
o Heart	- Heart failure (HF)
	- Atrial myxoma
o Lung	- Bronchiectasis
	- Abscess
	- Cancer
o Liver	- Cirrhosis
o Spleen	- Splenomegaly
o Nodes	- Lymphadenopathy
o MSK	- Rheumatoid arthritis
	- Lupus
o Malnutrition	

Adapted from: Jugovic PJ, et al. *Saunders/ Elsevier* 2004, pages 15 and 16.

- Give the performance characteristics of findings of anemia

Finding	PLR
o Conjunctival rim pallor	16.7
o Palmar crease pallor	7.9
o Palmar pallor	5.6
o Conjunctival pallor	4.7
o Pallor at any site	4.1
o Facial pallor (but not nail bed pallor)	3.8

Abbreviations: likelihood ratio (LR) if finding present= positive LR (PLR)

Adapted from: McGee SR. *Saunders/Elsevier* 2007, Box 8-1, page 91.

> What is "the best test for anemia"? The 'best test' for anemia is pallor in conjunctive, palms, face.

➤ Laboratory
  o Buzzwords
    - Sometimes on multiple choice questions (MCQs), certain terms are used to signal the presence of a particular diagnosis (part of the game of the examiner saying "guess what I'm thinking")

- For each of the following terms (often disguised in Latin or Greek), give the commonly associated hematological condition(s).

Buzzwords	Aka	Hematological conditions
o Acanthocytes	- Spur cells	Liver disease, severe
o Anisocytosis	- Microcytes	Iron deficiency
o Anisopoikilocytosis	- RBC size / shape variations	Iron deficiency
o Bile cells		G-6-PD deficiency
o Codocytes	- Large cells	Liver disease
		Splenectomy
		Hemoglobinopathy

Buzzwords	Aka	Hematological conditions
o Dacrocytes	- Tear drop cells	Bone marrow Infiltration Fibrosis Granuloma
o Deepanocytes	- Sickle cells	Sickle cell anemia
o Echinocytes	- Burr cells	Kidney disease
o Schistocytes		Microangiopathy

Adapted from MKSAP 16, Hematology and Oncology 2012; Table 10, page 18.

Useful definitions

➤ 'Tart cell
  o A monocyte or neutrophil which has phagocytosed another cell or nucleus.
  o Mimics the LE cell, but occurs in health and in disorders with raised immunoglobulins.

➤ Howell-Jolly bodies: Nuclear remnants seen as small dense purple particles at the periphery of RBCs
  o Causes
    - Splenectomy
    - Dyshemopoietic states: leukemia, megaloblastic anemia, etc

➤ Pappenheimer bodies: Fe-containing granules in siderocytes
  o Causes
    - Lead poisoning
    - Hemolytic anemia, which continues after splenectomy

➤ Heinz bodies: Peripheral rounded dark blue bodies in reticulocytes
  o Causes
    - Hemolytic anemia due to drugs and chemicals
    - Familial RBC defects (e.g. G6PD deficiency)
    - Rare hemoglobinopathies (e.g. Hb Koln) after splenectomy

➤ Causes of target cells
  o Iron
    - Iron deficiency anemia

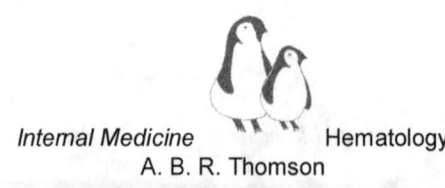

- o Hemolysis
  - Thalassemia
  - Sickle-cell anemia
- o Hemoglobin
  - Hemoglobin –C disease
- o Liver/spleen
  - Liver disease and obstructive jaundice
  - Splenectomy
- o Dehydration

Source: Burton JL. *Churchill Livingstone* 1971, page 52.

Pernicious Anemia

- Perform a focused physical examination for pernicious anemia.

  - o General
    - Middle age
    - Blue eyes
    - Hair
      - Blondish
      - Prematurely grey

  - o Signs of anemia

  - o CNS/PNS
    - Mental changes
    - ↓ position and vibration sensation (dorso-lateral column changes)
    - Peripheral neuropathy

  - o Eyes
    - Optic atrophy
    - Nystagmus

  - o Hepatosplenomegaly

  - o Causes of vitamin B12 deficiency
    - Lack of intrinsic factor
      - Pernicious anemia
      - Partial or total gastrectomy
    - Changed intestinal flora
      - Stricture
      - Blind-loop syndrome
      - Diverticulosis of small bowel
      - Fistulae

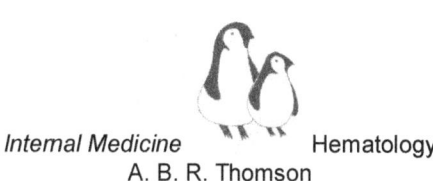

- Ileal damage
  - Crohn disease
  - Resection
- Parasites: Diphyllobothrium latum
- Dietary (rare)
- Pancreatitis (rare)

Abbreviations: UMN, upper motor neuron; LMN, lower motor neuron

Adapted from: Burton JL. *Churchill Livingstone* 1971, pages 57 and 58.

Macrocytic Anemia

- Give the causes of macrocytic anemia with normoblastic bone marrow.

  - Nutrition
    - Protein deficiency
    - Scurvy

  - White blood cell
    - Leukemia

  - Red blood cell
    - Hemolysis
    - Hemorrhage

  - Marrow
    - Aplastic anemia
    - Marrow infiltration or replacement

  - Liver
    - Cirrhosis

  - Endocrine
    - Myxedema or hypopituitarism

Adapted from: Burton JL. *Churchill Livingstone* 1971, page 25 and 58.

- Give 3 megaloblastic and 3 non-megaloblastic causes of macrocytic anemia.

  - Megaloblastic   - Deficiency of folate and/or cobalamin
    - Drugs affecting metabolism of folate and / or cobalamin
    - Myelodysplastic syndromes

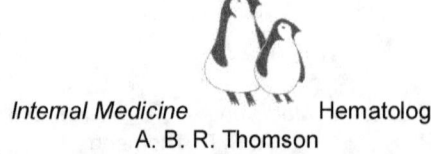

Internal Medicine   Hematology
A. B. R. Thomson

o   Non-megaloblastic   -   Chronic liver disease
                         -   Hyposplenism / asplenia
                         -   Reticulocytosis

In the patient with suspected hemolytic anemia (anemia, ↑ reticulocyte count; ↑ MCV if ↑ reticulocytes, ↑ LDH, ↑ indirect bilirubin, ↓ haptogloblin), the Coombs test is reported to be positive.

- Give the meaning of the Coombs test, and the meaning of positive Coombs test regarding the cause of hemolysis.

    o   The Coombs test   -   A direct anti-globulin test to detect IgG or complement on the surface of RBCs

    o   A positive   -   Indicates that the hemolysis in immune-
        Coombs test   mediated

CLINICAL PEARL AND GEMS

o   Don't make your patient suffer with vitamin B12 injections, when they can easily replenish their body stores of cobalamin by using intranasal or oral (tablets, gels) treatment.

o   In the presence of severe cobalamin deficiency, start low dose replacement therapy, and consider giving supplements of folate and iron because of their impending rapid demand in response to the ↑ erythrocytosis.

o   In the person with folate deficiency and a low serum folate concentration, one hardy meal o leafy green vegetables and bananas may be sufficient to correct the low folate concentration, so measure RBC folate on first encounter

o   "Alcohol" (i.e., ethanol) intake can cause macrocytosis and low serum folate concentrations, so either routinely use folic acid supplements, or prove deficiency with ↓ RBC folate and then supplement

o   All patients with hemolytic anemia require daily supplements of folic acid.

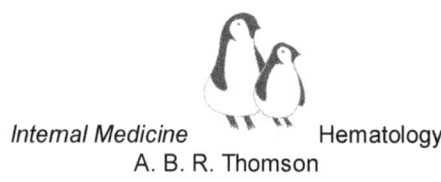

Internal Medicine   Hematology
A. B. R. Thomson

Polycythemia

➢ Causes

• Absolute

➢ Primary (please see previous section polycythemia vera (PV)

➢ Secondary
  o Hypoxic
    - Intake
      ▪ High altitude (Monge's disease)
      ▪ Cerebral (decreased respiratory drive)
      ▪ Obesity
    - Circulation
      ▪ Cardiac or pulmonary disease
    - Blinding
      ▪ Methemoglobinemia and sulphemoglobinemia
  o ↑ Erythropoietin
    - CNS
      ▪ Hemagiomas
      ▪ Cerebellar hemangioblastoma
    - Kidney disease
    - Lung bronchial cancer
    - Liver
      ▪ Carcinoma of liver (HCC)
    - GU
      ▪ Uterine myomata
      ▪ Ovarian tumors

  ➢ Endocrine
    o Adrenal cancer/hyperplasia
    o Pheochromocytoma

• Relative
  o Dehydration
  o 'Stress' polycythemia

Adapted from: Burton JL. *Churchill Livingstone* 1971, page 62.

  ➢ CNS
    o Hemangiomas

  ➢ Lung
    o Bronchial cancer

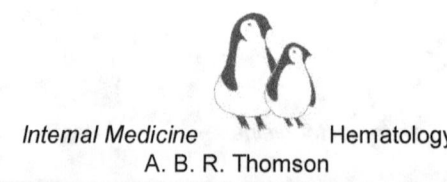

> Kidney
>> o   Renal cancer
>> o   Benign tumors

Adapted from: Burton JL. *Churchill Livingstone* 1971, page 62.

Hypochromic Anemia

It may be difficult to distinguish between iron deficiency anemia and inflammatory anemia, such as in the patient with Crohn disease. Both will have ↓ serum iron concentration and ↓ TS (transferrin saturation; sometimes the TS may be normal in inflammatory anemia). Both may be normocytic or microcytic (curiously, about a third of patients with iron deficiency will have a normal MCV).

- Give the differences between iron deficiency (FeD) and anemia of chronic disease (ACD).

Cell type	FeD	ACD
o Normochronic, normocytic, or hypochromin, microcytic	+	+
o Anisocytosis	+	-
o Reticulocyte count	↑	↓
o Serum iron	N / ↓	N / ↓
o TIBC	↑	↓↓
o Ferritin	↓	↑
o Fe in bone marrow	0	N / ↑
o IL-1, IL-6, interferon	N	↑
o Hepcidin	↓	↑

Abbreviations: Fe, iron; TIBC, total iron-binding capacity; N, normal

* Note: if the patient has inflammatory anemia and the serum ferritin concentration is > 100 ng/mL, then they do not have associated iron deficiency

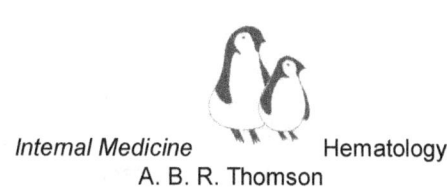

Internal Medicine   Hematology
A. B. R. Thomson

➢ Causes
  o ↓ intake of folate, cobalamin (mixture of macrocytes and normocytes)
  o ↓ production
    - ↓ erythropoietin
    - ↓ metabolism
    - Hypothyroidism
    - Testosterone deficiency

  o ↓ release of iron inflammatory blockage (inflammatory anemia, aka anemia of chronic disease)
  o Ideopathic

Aplastic Anemia

➢ Causes
  o Idiopathic
  o Drugs, chemicals (e.g., iodine)

➢ Clinical

• Give the typical clinical presentation of the patient with aplastic anemia.

  o ↓ RBC   -   Fatigue

  o ↓ WBC   -   Fever

  o ↓ platelets   -   Nose bleeds

➢ Laboratory

• Give the diagnostic tests for pure red cell aplasia (PRCA).

  o PRCA is diagnosed from
    - CD57+ T-cells on flow cytometry
    - Clonality on T-cell receptor gene rearrangement studies

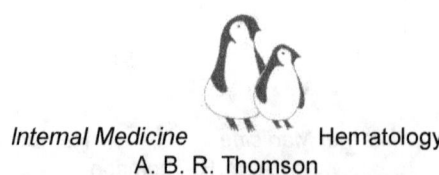

Internal Medicine   Hematology
A. B. R. Thomson

- Give 2 conditions causing aplastic anemia which can be diagnosed on flow cytometry.
  - Lack of expression of CD55 or CD59 on RBC
    - PNH (paroxysmal nocturnal hemoglobulinuria)
  - Monoclonal CD57-positive T cell population
    - Acquired chronic red cell aplasia

- Give 2 hematological complications of a parvovirus B19 infection in the patient with HIV / AIDs.
  - Chronic pure red cell aplasia
  - Transient aplastic crisis in the patient with sickle cell disease

---

CLINICALGEM

  - The patient with a mechanical heart valve who develops microangiopathic hemolytic anemia from intravascular hemolysis from chemotherapeutic regimens requires an echocardiogram to detect
    - Valvular regurgitation
    - Paravalvular leakage

Sideroblastic Anemia

➤ Pathology
  - Iron accumulates in RBC precursors

➤ Causes of sideroblastic anemia
  - Hypochromic anemia with large numbers of normoblasts containing many iron granules in the marrow
  - Congenital (Pseudo-thalassemia)
  - Refractory normoblastic anemia of adults
  - Lead poisoning
  - Nutritional
    - B_{12}, folate deficiency, pyridoxine (INH therapy)

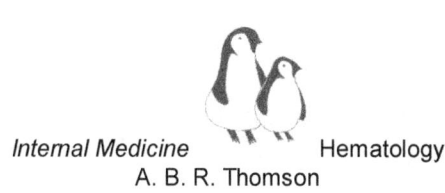

Internal Medicine   Hematology
A. B. R. Thomson

➤ Miscellaneous blood dyscrasias

- o Myeloproliferative disease

- o Myelomatosis

- o Collagen disease

- o Carcinoma

Adapted from: Burton JL. *Churchill Livingstone* 1971, page 53.

Sickle Cell Anemia

➤ Definition

- o Sickle cell disease is a systemic, multiple organ disease which is caused by a point mutation and single amino acid substitution at the 6th position of the β-globin chain and leads to disease which includes phenotype diversity within a given genotype

- o Sickling Syndrome
  - Co-inheritance
    - Hb D plus HbS
    - HbE plus β-thalassemia

➤ Clinical

- o General
  - Vaso-occlusive pain
  - Thromboembolism
  - ↑ risk of infection
  - Multi-organ failure

- o CNS
  - Ischemic stroke
  - Retinopathy

- o CVS
  - Sudden death

- o Lung
  - Acute chest syndrome
  - Pulmonary hypertension

- o Bone
  - Infarcts
  - Osteonecrosis

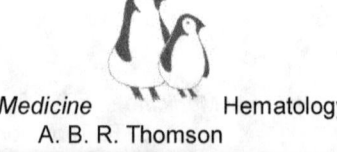

Internal Medicine   Hematology
A. B. R. Thomson

- o GI
  - Hepatopathy
  - Gallstones
- o GU
  - CKI (chronic kidney insufficiency)
  - Priapism
  - Renal medullary carcinoma

- o Blood
  - Anemia
  - Aplastic crisis (precipitation by infection with parvovirus B19)
  - Delayed hemolytic transfusion reaction
  - Splenic rupture

- o Skin
  - Ulceration

- o MSK
  - Aches and pain
  - Needs to rule out veno-occlusive disease

➢ Management
  - o Ensure correct diagnosis

  - o Supportive care
    - Hydration
    - Analgesia
    - O_2 therapy
    - Genetic counseling

  - o Hydroxyurea
    - Veno-oclusive pain episodes
      - Morphine, hydromorphone
      - Patient controlled analgesia (PCA)
      - NSAIDs
    - Acute chest syndrome
    - Anemia, symptomatic
    - ↓ Mortality rate

    - ≥ 2 pain episodes per year
    - ACS
    - No hydroxyurea during pregnancy (teratogenic; stop at least 3 mon before planned pregnancy)

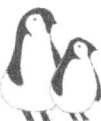

- o Transfusions
  - Ischemic stroke (CVA)
  - Acute chest syndrome (ACS)
  - Symptomatic anemia
  - Surgery
  - RBC for transfusion in SC disease
    - Leuko reduced
    - Hbs negative
    - Matched for E, C, Kell antigens
  - Matched for known alloantibodies
  - Target hemoglobin < 10 g/dL to avoid hyperviscosity
  - Chelation therapy for associated hemosiderosis

- In the context of sickle of sickle cell disease, give the meaning of the "Moyamoya syndrome".
  - o Moyamoya syndrome
    - Formation of collateral vasculature due to
      - Vasculopathy
      - Neovascularization

- Give the precautions to be taken in the sickle cell patient who requires a blood transfusion.

  - o To avoid DHTR
    - Target hemoglobin concentration (Hb) – 100 g/L (10 g/dL)
    - Phenotypic matching of RBC for CCK antigens any other antigens to which there is alloantibody

  - o To avoid venoocclusion
    - Hb-S negative blood

  - o To avoid GVHD
    - Irradiation of RBC

Abbreviation: DHTR, delayed hemolytic transfusion reaction

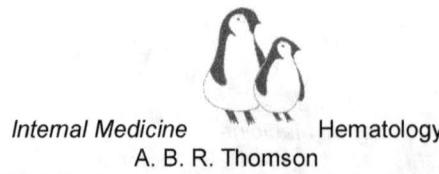

o EET (RBC exchange transfusion)
  - Ischemic stroke (CVA)
  - Acute chest syndrome (ACS)
  - Pulmonary hypertension
  - Hepatopathy
  - Multi-organ failure
  - Priapism
  - Symptomatic chronic anemia
  - Aplastic crisis
  - Skin ulcers
  - Therapeutic
    Acute CVA
    Fat embolism
  - Prophylactic
    History of ischemic CVA

o Aspirin
  - Ischemic stroke

o O_2, incentive spasmetry
  - ACS bronchodilators

o Empiric antibiotics
  - ACS
  - Associated infection
  - Target Hb > 100 g/L (10 g/dL)

o Joint replacement
  - Osteonecrosis

o Erythropoietin
  - Severe anemia
  - Chronic renal disease

CLINICAL GEM

Persons infected with parvovirus B19 often have fever, arthralgias and ↓ reticulocyte count

---

Internal Medicine   Hematology
A. B. R. Thomson

➢ Laboratory

• From the reticulocyte count, differentiate between 3 causes of sudden worsening of anemia in patients with sickle cell disease.

	Cause	Reticulocyte count
Aplastic crisis	Parvovirus B19 infection	↓
Megaloblastic crisis	Folate deficiency	↓
Hyperhemolytic crisis	Unknown	↑

• Give the laboratory methods to diagnosis parvovirus B19 infection.

   o IgM antibodies against parvovirus B19

   o PCR (polymerase chain reaction) detection of parvovirus B19 DNA

   o When persons with sickle cell anemia become infected with parvovirus B19, there is ↓ production of RBCs and aplastic crisis

   o In hereditary spherocytosis, parvovirus B19 may also cause a transient aplastic crisis

➢ Differential

• Sickle cell disease is a greater mimicker. Give the manner in which sickle cell disease is differentiated from

   o Lung   - Pneumonia
                                  ▪ Diffuse rather than localized infiltration
                               - Fat embolus
                                  ▪ Fat bodies in bronchial washings or sputum
                               - Pulmonary embolus
                                  ▪ CT chest / angiography gives different pattern

   o Gallbladder   - Cholecystitis vs. hepatic crisis
                                  ▪ Abdominal ultrasound will exclude bilirubin stones
                                  ▪ ↑↑transaminases in ischemic hepatitis

o Simple anemia of Sickle cell disease vs. aplastic crisis or hyperhemolysis

- In crisis
  - ↓ Hg ≥ 2 g/dL

- Aplastic crisis
  - Cytotoxic drugs, parvovirus B19, idiopathic
  - Reticulocyte count ↓

- Hyperhemolysis
  - ↑ bilirubin, ↑ LDH, ↑ transaminases
  - Reticulocyte count ↑
  - Mycoplasma infection
  - Transfusion reaction
  - Associated reaction
  - Associated G6P deficiency

o RLQ sickle cell pain vs. appendicitis
  - Fever, tenderness, pain, ↓ bowel sounds, ↑ WBC → Appendicitis
  - ↑ LDH, normal bowel sounds → Sickle cell disease

• Give a simple laboratory test which helps to confirm that a patient with sickle cell anemia is adhering to the recommendation to take their hydroyurea treatment.

o An ↑ MCV (mean cell volume) suggests that this RNA-reductase inhibitor (hydroxyurea) is being taken.

o Team approach because of ↑ mortality for
  - Homozygous SS ~ 2%
  - Compound heterozygotes (5 plus B-thalassemia or HbC) ~ 1% trait – normal complication rate

o Complications
  - ↑ mortality
  - Menarche later
  - First pregnancy later
  - ↑ fetal loss
  - ↑ number of low-birth weight neonates

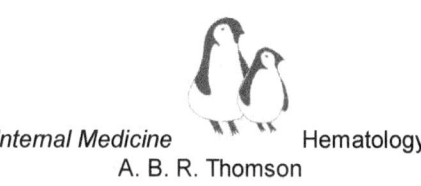

➢ Treatment

In the patient with sickle cell disease who is known to have alloantibodies and who needs a blood transfusion, give the way in which the risk may be reduced of a DHTR (delayed hemolytic transfusion reaction).

    o Transfuse phenotypically matched RBCs

Acute Chest Syndrome

➢ Definition
    o Dyspnea

    o Fever

    o Hypoxia

    o New infiltrate in chest X-ray (usually on entire lung segment)

➢ Causes
    o Infection

    o Infarction

    o Infiltration: fat embolization

• Give the treatment of acute chest syndromes In the context of sickle cell disease

    o IV hydration (do not over hydrate)

    o O_2

    o RBC transfusion if hypoxia persists

    o Exchange transfusion if hypoxia still persists

    o Bronchodilators for patients with reactive airway disease

    o Incentive spirometry

    o Pain control

    o Empiric antibiotics

    o Avoid overhydration

    o Note – hydroxyurea is useful for long-term management to ↓ risk of acute chest syndrome, but is **not** of use in the acute setting.

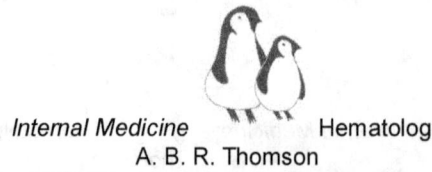

- Give 2 treatments which ↓ risk of ACS (acute chest syndrome).

  - Outpatient   -   Hydroxyurea

  - Inpatient   -   Incentive spirometry

- Give the reason why meperidine is not a first choice analgesic for pain arising from sickle cell crisis.

  - Meperidine is metabolized to normeperidine
  - Normaperidine accumulates as a toxic metabolite
  - Normeperidine lowers the seizure threshold
  - Hemoglobin electrophoresis allows for identification of the abnormal hemoglobin which arises from single-base substitution of the B gene
  - Hemolytic arises and aplastic crisis may arise from parvovirus B19 infection
  - Deformed sickle RBCs block small vessels, and thereby cause disease.

Pearls and Gems

- Give the reason why opioids are preferred over meperidine to treat the pain of a sickle cell crisis.
  - The metabolic product of meperidine is normeperidine
  - If normeperidine accumulated, the patient may have a seizure

- Give the contraindications of the use of hydroxyurea.
  - Pregnancy
  - Renal failure

Patients with chronic hemolytic anemia require daily supplements of folic acid, as well as periodic RBC transfusions.

- Give specific therapies for 5 causes of hemolytic anemia.

    o Plasma exchange — TTP

    o HSCT
    - Severe thalassemia
    - Severe PNH
    - Autoimmune hemolytic anemia not responding to corticosteroids

    o Splenectomy*
    - Hereditary spherocytosis
    - Transfusion-dependent thalassemia

    o Autoimmune hemolytic anemia (warm-body and cold agglutinin) corticosteroids → splenectomy → immune suppression, immune globulin, rituximab, danazol

Abbreviations: HSCT, human stem cell transplantation; PNH, paroxysmal nocturnal hemoglobinuria; TTP, thrombocytopenic purpura thrombotic

*Note:
- o Vaccinations are needed before splenectomy

- o These vaccinations include
    - Pneumococcus
    - Haemophillus influenza type B
    - Influenza
    - Meningococcus

Tricks and Red Herrings

A low Glucose-6-phosphate dehydrogenase (G-6-PD) deficiency may cause hemolytic anemia.

- Give the time when the G-6-PD activity may be normal and lead to a false-negative test result for G-6-PD deficiency.

    o During an acute hemolytic episode, the G-6-PD level may be normal
    o Wait 2-3 mon after an acute hemolytic episode to measure G-6-PD activity to attempt to diagnose G-6-PD deficiency.

HEMOLYSIS

Hemolytic Anemias

- Give 4 clues from screening blood tests that an anemia is hemolytic in origin.

    o ↑ reticulocytes, indirect bilirubin, lactate dehydrogenase; hemoglobinuria

    o ↓ haptoglobulin

- Conditions to be considered here

➤ Congenital
    o Hereditary spherocytosis
    o Glucose-6-phosphate dehydrogenase (G-6-PD) deficiency
    o Thalassemia syndrome
    o Sickle cell syndrome

➤ Acquired
    o Autoimmune
    o Warm autoimmune
    o Cold agglutinin disease
    o Microangiopathic
    o Paroxysmal nocturnal hemoglobinuria (PHN)

➤ Clinical

- Take a directed history for causes of hemolytic anemia.

    o Paroxysmal nocturnal hemoglobinuria
    o Hemolytic disease of the newborn
      - Rhesus
      - ABO

    o Inherited
      - Hereditary spherocytosis, elliptocytosis
      - Hereditary non- spherocytic anemia
      - Thalassemia and Thal. like disorders
      - Sickle-cell disease and S.C disease - like hemoglobinopathies

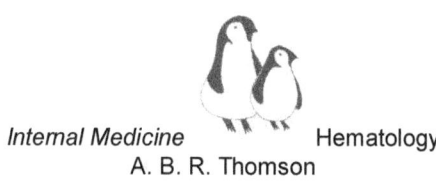

- o Immune
  - Idiopathic (warm or cold antibodies)
  - Viral or mycoplasma infection
  - Paroxysmal cold hemoglobinuria (syphilitic or non-syphilitic)

- o Infiltration
  - Hematological
    - Malignant disease of lympho-reticular system
  - Solid
    - Myeloproliferative disorders
    - Carcinomatosis
    - Ovarian tumors
    - Atrial myxoma

- o Infections
  - Bacterial
    - Coccal septicaemia
    - Clostridium welchii
    - Oroya fever
    - TB
    - Typhoid
    - 'H.influenzae' meningitis
  - Protozoal
    - Malaria (Blackwater fever)
    - Kala-azar

- o Renal
  - Chronic renal failure
  - 'Hemolytic-uraemia' syndrome (infants and children)
  - Thrombotic thrombocytopaenic purpura (TTP)
  - Malignant hypertension
  - Eclampsia, or post-partum

- o Pregnancy

- o Endocrine disease
  - Myxedema
  - Hypopituitarism
  - Hypoadrenalism

- o Hypersplenism

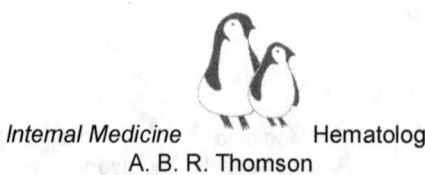

o Liver disease	- Hepatitis
	- Cirrhosis
o Inflammatory	- Crohn disease, ulcerative colitis
o Immune	- SLE
o Nutritional	- Protein deficiency
	- Scurvy
	- Megaloblastic anemia
o Trauma	- Cardiac surgery
	- March hemoglobinuria'
	- Burns
	- Radiation

Adapted from: Burton JL. *Churchill Livingstone* 1971, page 54.

Hereditary Spherocytosis

➢ Demography
  o 50 / 10^5 Northern Europeans
  o Autosomal dominant with penetrance, or sporatic

➢ Pathophysiology
  o Mutations in anchoring proteins, such as ankyrin, lead to destabilized spherocytic cells
  o May be associated with an aplastic crisis when there is an associated parvovirus 19 infection

➢ Diagnosis
  o Negative direct Coombs test
  o Positive osmotic fragility test

➢ Treatment
  o Vaccination
    - Pneumococcus Meningococcus
      ▪ H. influenza type B
    - Splenectomy

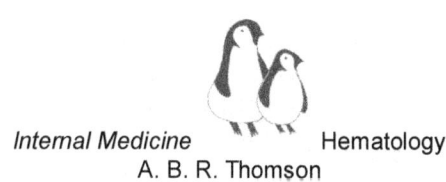

Paroxysmal Nocturnal Hemoglobulinuria (PNH)

➢ Definition
  o Clonal stem cell disorder associated with mutations in PIG-A gene which lead to
    - ↓ glycosylphosphatidylinositol (GPPI)
    - ↓ CD 55 (decay-accelerating factor) ⎤ GPPI-dependent complement
    - ↓ CD59 (membrane inhibitor of active lysis) ⎦ regulatory protein
  o Result in thrombosis in vascular beds such as cerebral and mesenteric

➢ Clinical

• Give the clinical presentation of PNH (paroxysmal nocturnal hemoglobulinuria).

  o Iron deficiency (from hemoglobulinuria)
  o Hemolytic anemia
  o Pancytopenia (end aplasia)
  o Venous thrombosis (include venous thrombosis of mesenteric vessels)

➢ Treatment
  o Transfusion of RBC
  o Immunosuppression plus anti-thymocytic globulin and cyclosporine
  o Eculizumab
  o Anticoagulation
  o HSCT (human stem cell transplantation)
  o Anti-coagulation
  o Iron and folic acid

  o Thrombotic events
    - Acute   Anti-coagulate
    - Preventive   Anti-coagulation if > 50% of RBC are deficient in CD 55 or CD 59

- o Vaccination for meningococcus, followed by
  - Eculizumab
  - Immunosuppression
  - Allogenic bone marrow transplantation
- o Severe unresponsive hemolytic or aplastic anemia
  - Corticosteroids
  - Iron
  - Erythropoietin

➢ Prognosis

- o ↑ mortality rate from
  - Thromboembolism
  - Progressive pancytopenia

CLINICAL PEARL AND GEMS

- o The presence of anemia, microcytosis, ↓ SI, ↓ % TIBC saturation, ↓ ferritin and ↑ sTR and ↓ hepcidin, suggests iron deficiency anemia

  - In "anemia of chronic disease" (aka inflammatory anemia), there may be no obviously associated inflammatory process, but remember that the inflammatory cytokines (IL-6, IL-1, interferon) are increased in chronic heart failure and diabetes

  - If the hemoglobin concentration is < 8 g/dL, the anemia is probably not sTR from a chronic disease association

  - sTR is usually normal in inflammatory anemia, and there is usually stainable iron in the bone marrow

  - RDW may be normal in inflammatory anemia and, ↑ in iron deficiency

Abbreviation: PNH, paroxysmal nocturnal hemoglobinuria; RBC, red blood cell

---

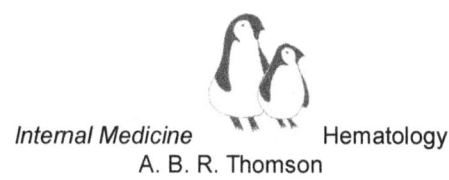

Glucose-6-Phosphate dehydrogenase (G-6-PD) **Deficiency**

➢ Definition

  o Mutation in X chromosome leads to inability of RBC to produce NADPH (nicotinamide adenosine dinucleotide phosphate), which is necessary to maintain glutathione in a reduced state.

➢ Clinical

  o African American variant
    - Acute hemolysis in response to oxidant stressors to
      ▪ Infection
      ▪ Drugs
        - Dapsone
        - Trimethoprime-sulfamethoxazole
        - Nitrofurantoin
    - Peripheral smear
      ▪ Bite RBC
      ▪ Heinz bodies

DIAGNOSTIC CAUTION

":...elevated levels of G-6-PD are found in young reticulocytes [in the African American variant], and G-6-PD levels may therefore be falsely normal during a hemolytic episode" (MKSAP 16, Hematology and Oncology, 2012, page 27)

To assess safety of drugs in persons with G-6-PD deficiency, please refer to

www.g6pd.org/favism/english/index.mvc?pgid=safe

Thalassemia

➢ Definition

  o Abnormal synthesis or either α- or β-chains in hemoglobin, leading to abnormal hemoglobin tetrameric structure, and therefore ineffective erythropoiesis as well as hemolytic anemia with target cells.

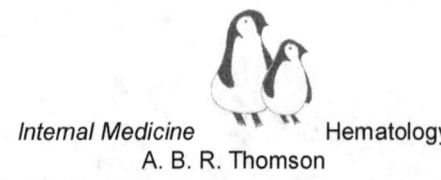

➢ Types

  ○ Two gene mutations lead to a trait, e.g. Thalassemia α- or β- minor

  ○ Deletion of 3α genes → hemoglobin disease

  ○ Deletion of 4α genes (homozygous inheritance of double gene deletion) → hydrops fetalis (- - / -)

  ○ Involvement of αβ chains → β-thalassemia trait (minor),
    - May have ↑ hemoglobin A2 and F

  ○ Deletion of 4β genes → β-thalassemia major (aka Cooley anemia)

  ○ Thalassemia intermedia ↓ but not absent β chain

  ○ Hb 5α thalassemia may mimic sickle cell disease

• In the context of Thalassemia, give the meaning of the Mentzer Index and its significance.

  ○ Mentzer Index: MCV / RBC count

  ○ When MCV / RBC < 13, suspect β-thalassemia

α-thalassemia trait (minor, - α / - α, or - - / αα) may be mistaken for iron deficiency, especially when the hemoglobin electrophoresis is normal.

• Give the use if RDW to distinguish thalassemia minor from iron deficiency.

Condition	RDW
Iron deficiency	↑
Thalassemia	Normal

• There are many causes of microcytic anemia. Without having access to the chemical nature of a patient's hemoglobin B-chain (↓ B-chain synthesis → ↓ Hb (hemoglobin) A [α2β2], and increased HbA^2 or HbF, give a way to predict that a patient has β-thalassemia trait.

  ○ In B-thalassemia trait, there is a microtic anemia plus ↑ RBC count.

  ○ This is reflected in the Mentzer index: MCV (mean cell volume) /RBC

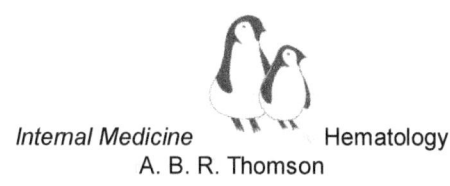

Internal Medicine   Hematology
A. B. R. Thomson

- o When the Mentzer index < 13, there is a strong possibility of B-thalassemia.

A normal hemoglobin electrophoresis does not exclude the diagnosis of α-thalassemia trait.

- Give the name of the laboratory test to make the definitive diagnosis.

  - o Studies of the globin gene synthesis

- ➢ Treatment
  - o Life-long regular RBC transfusions
  - o Treatment of associated iron overload (from breakdown of transfused RBCs)
  - o Splenectomy (↓ RBC destruction in spleen, so ↓ RBC transfusion requirements)
  - o HSCT (curative)

THERAPEUTIC CHALLENGE

The iron overload from multiple transfusions from B-thalassemia but not hereditary hemochromatosis is treated with iron chelation deferasirox.

- Give the reason for the differential but not the iron overload from hereditary hemochromatosis (HH),

  - o When thalassemia is transfusion-dependent, the patient needs the oxygen-carrying capacity of the transfused blood, whereas in HH the phlebotomy is undertaken to remove the excess body iron while the patient's hemoglobin concentration remains unchanged.

AUTOIMMUNE HEMOLYTIC ANEMIAS (AIHA)

- ➢ Types
  - o Warm autoimmune hemolytic anemia (WAIHA)
  - o Cold agglutinin disease (CAD)

- ➢ Associations
  - o Inflammation
    - Autoimmune conditions
  - o Infiltration
    - Malignancy
    - Lymphoproliferative disorders
  - o Infection
  - o Iatrogenic
    - Drugs / chemicals

- ➢ Laboratory
  - o Antibodies
    - IgG, 80%
    - IgM, 20%

- Give the anticipated results of the direct Coombs (anti-globulin) test in the patient with suspected warm autoimmune hemolytic anemia.
  - o The direct Coombs
    - Strongly positive   ▪ IgG
    - Weakly positive   ▪ Complement

Warm Autoimmune Hemolytic Anemia

- ➢ Pathogenesis
  - o IgG antibiotics bind to Rh antigens at 37 °C, and these IgG antibody-coated RBCs bind to Fc receptors on macrophages in spleen, resulting in partial phagocytosis of RBC membrane, and formation of spherocytes.

➢ Diagnosis	WAIHA	B small cell clone	CAD	RBC shape	Antibody	Macrophage binding
o Direct Coombs test	+ IgG	+	+	Spherocytes	IgG	Spleen
o C3 (complement)	+ in 10%					

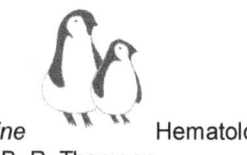

➤ Tratment

    o Prednisone

    o For prednisone non-responders
- Azathioprine
- Cyclosporine
- Cyclophosphamide
- Danazol
- Rituximab
- Splenectomy

Cold Agglutinin Disease (CAD)

➤ Pathogenesis
    o IgM antibody binds in the cold to RBC membrane, and fixes complement, resulting in RBC cleared by
- Binding to macrophages in liver
- Intravascular lysis

SO YOU WANT TO BE A HEPATOLOGIST!

- Give the explanation for the ↑ risk of acute or delayed hemolytic transfusion reaction in CAD.
  - The IgM antibody titre may become high in warmed blood
  - Alloantibodies may be masked and not detected by the blood bank service technicians.

- In the context of CAD (cold agglutinin disease, with RBC hemolysis), give the name of the 2 common infections which may be associated with CAD during the patient's convalescence.
  - Mycoplasma
  - EBV (Epstein-Barr Virus)

- Give the explanation for the increased mean cell volume (↑ MCV) which occurs in CAD (cold agglutinin disease).
  - No, the ↑ MCV is not from
    - Alcohol
    - Liver disease
    - Deficiency of folate and vitamin B12
    - Reticulocytosis
  - In CAD, the RBC are clumped together, so that they are mistaken to be big cells with large volumes, but they are simply agglutinated RBC.

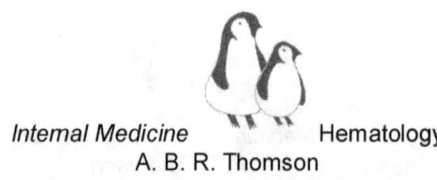

➢ Treatment

  o Acute disease　　- Plasmapheresis

  o Chronic
  - Chloambucil
  - Cyclophosphamide
  - Rituximab

  o RBC transfusion
  - Cautious use of warmed blood

  o Keep the body warm

Microangiopathic Hemolytic Anemia

➢ Definition

  o Passage of RBC through the vascular system cases fragmentation of the cells, the formation of schistocytes (helmet cells), and intravascular hemolysis.

➢ Causes (examples)

  o Macrovascular
  - Damaged mechanical heart valve
  - Intra-aortic balloon

  o Microvascular
  - Hemolytic uremic syndrome (HUS)
  - Thrombocytopenic purpura (TTP)
  - Disseminated intravascular coagulopathy)

  o Pregnancy and liver disease
  - HELLP syndrome
  - Pre-eclampsia

  o Kidney
  - Scleroderma renal crisis

  o CVS
  - Hypertension
  - Vasculitis

➢ Treatment

  o Treat the underlying condition

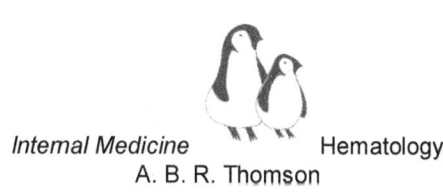

- ○ Plasma exchange for TTP / HUS

- ○ Treat associated iron deficiency

- ○ Erythropoietin when anemias symptomatic and underlying disease does not respond to treatment

- ○ Drugs

- ○ Malignancy

Buzzwords, trivia, and ridiculous MCQs

If the clinical stem is that of a patient with hemolytic anemia and one of the following phrases, watch out: forewarned is forearmed

Watch out for	They are thinking about
○ Travel to Cape Cod, Nantucket Island or Northern California	- Babesiosis
○ Travel to Indonesia, Malaysia	- Malaria
○ Travel to South America	- Bartonellosis
○ Works in battery factory	- Arsine gas
○ Young person with jaundice, behavioural problems, renal tubular acidosis, Kayser-Fleisher rings	- Wilson disease (copper-induced hemolysis)

WHITE BLOOD CELLS

- • Give the causes of eosinophilia (>440/cu.mm.)

  - ○ Allergy

  - ○ Infection: Hookworms, tapeworm, hydatid, ascaris, bilharzias, strongyloides, filarial, trichina, Post-infectious rebound

  - ○ Drugs: penicillin, streptomycin, chlorpromazine

  - ○ Skin diseases
    - - Scabies
    - - Dermatitis herpetiformis
    - - Atopic eczema
    - - Erythema neonatorum

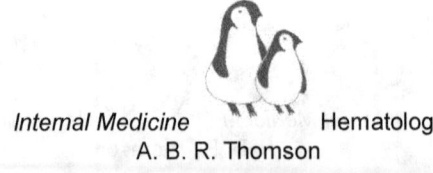

- o Pulmonary eosinophilia
  - Asthma (including aspergillosis)
  - Polyarteritis nodosa
  - Tropical eosinophilia
  - Loeffler's

- o Hematological
  - Blood dyscrasias (including eosinophilic leukemia)

- o Tumor
  - Malignancy

- o Miscellenous
  - Eosinophilic granuloma

- o Gastrophilic syndromes
  - Post splenectomy
  - Eosinophilic gastroenteritis

Adapted from: Burton JL. *Churchill Livingstone* 1971, page 61.

- Give the causes of pancytopenia / neutropenia.

  - o Marrow infiltration

  - o Hypersplenism

  - o Deficiency
    - Megaloblastic anemia
    - Iron deficient anemia

  - o PNH (paroxysmal nocturnal hemoglobinuria)

  - o Endocrine
    - Hypo-/hyperthyroidism
    - Cirrhosis

  - o Immune
    - Lupus

- ➢ Causes of neutropenia

  - o Infection
    - Viral
    - Chronic bacterial,

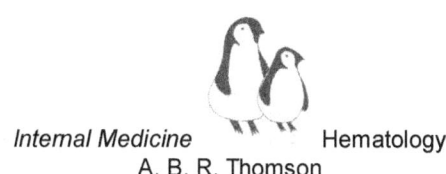

- o Malignancy infiltration
    - Carcinomatous metastasis to bone
    - Myelosclerosis
    - Myeloma
    - Malignant lymphoma
- o Non-malignant infiltration
    - Gauchers
    - Niemann-Picks
    - Histiocytosis X

Neutropenia

Congenital Asymptomatic Neutropenia

➢ Definition

- o Absolute neutrophil count (ANC) between 1.0 to 1.5 x 10^9 /L (1000 to 1500 /µL)

➢ Demographics common in

- o Africans

- o Jews, Yemenites

- o Arabs, especially Jordanian

➢ No complications; no therapy needed

Febrile Neutropenia

Febrile neutropenia is a medical emergency. After taking blood and urine samples for culture, empiric antibiotics must be started immediately.

- Give the recommended immediate empiric therapy for febrile neutropenia.

- o Piperracillin-tazobactam (penicillin / β-lactamase inhibitor, plus

- o Cefepime (3rd –generation cephalosporin)

Minocytosis

➢ Causes

• Give the causes of monocytosis (>800/cu.mm).

 o Infectious
   - Viral –infectious mononucleosis
   - Rickettsial- Rocky Mountain spotted fever
   - Bacterial- Listeria monocytogenes
   - TB
   - Brucellosis
   - Typhoid
   - Subacute bacterial endocarditis (SBE)
   - Protozoal - Malaria, kala-azar, trypanosomiasis

 o Malignancy
   - Hodgkin's disease
   - Monocytic leukemia

Leukocytosis

➢ Causes (>10,000/cu.mm in adults)
 o Physiological
   - Infancy
   - Pregnancy and post-partum

 o Infection

 o Hemorrhage

 o Trauma, burns, surgery

 o Myocardial infarction and paroxysmal tachycardia

 o Toxins: steroids, digitalis, adrenaline, lead, mercury, carbon monoxide

 o Collagen vascular diseases

 o Infiltration
   – Tumor
   – Myeloproliferative disorders

 o Metabolic disorders: renal failure, gout, diabetic coma, eclampsia

 o Miscellaneous
   - Hemolysis
   - Serum. Sickness
   - Acute anoxia
   - Spider venom

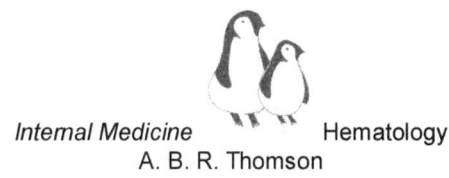

Internal Medicine　　　Hematology
A. B. R. Thomson

- Give the causes of **myeloid leukamoid reaction** (WCC>50,000/ cu.mm or myelocytes or myeloblasts present in peripheral blood).

  o Infections

  o Malignancy

  o Acute hemolysis

  o Leuco-erythroblastic anemia
    - Marble bone disease (Albers-Schonberg)

- Give the causes of **lymphocytosis** (>3500/cu.mm).

  o Infections
    - Viral: infectious mononucleosis; infective hepatitis; infectious lymphocytosis, influenza, exanthemata
    - Bacterial: pyogenic infections in young children, convalescence from acute infections, pertussis, typhoid, brucellosis, TB, Syphilis
    - Protozoal: toxoplasmosis

  o Infiltration
    - Lymphatic leukemia
    - Carcinoma
    - Myeloma

  o Endocrine
    - Myasthenia gravis
    - Thyrotoxicosis
    - Hypopituitarism
  o Physiological (in early childhood)

- Give the causes of **agranulocytosis**.

  o Drugs

  o Aplastic anemia

  o Leukemia in subleukemic phase

  o Hypersplenism

  o Idiopathic

Adapted from: Burton JL. *Churchill Livingstone* 1971, pages 59 to 61.

LEUKEMIA

To be covered here:

- o Chronic lymhocytic
- o Hairy cell
- o Acute lymphoplastic
- o Acute myeloid

- A patient with acute leukemia has > 25% blasts cells in the bone marrow. Give the way a cell line can be diagnosed, and the appropriate therapy.

  - o Lymphocyte lineage may be diagnosed as lymphoid based on the markers
    - B-cell   CD10+, CD20+
    - T cell   TdT+

  - o Induction therapy
    - Anthracycline
    - L-asparaginase
    - Corticosteroids
    - Vincristine

Chronic Lymphocytic Leukemia (CLL)

- ➢ Types
  - o B cell CLL   -   Western countries
  - o T cell CLL   -   Asian counties
- ➢ Clinical stages
  - o ↑ lymphocytes, no symptoms

    | I | Lymphadenopathy |
    | II | Splenomegaly |
    | III | Anemia |
    | IV | Thrombocytopenia |

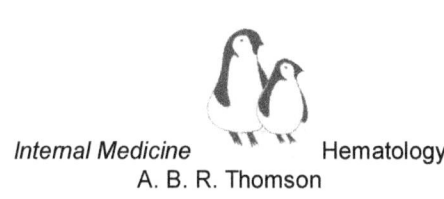

➢ Diagnosis and prognosis

• Give tests used to establish the prognosis of CLL.

  ○ Clinical stage
  ○ Lymphocyte doubling time
  ○ Serum B2-macroglobulin concentration
  ○ Immunophenotyping
  ○ Cytogenic studies
  ○ FISH (fluorescence in situ hybridization) testing
  ○ Mutational gene

➢ Treatment
  ○ Indications   - Symptoms, or
                                   - Poor prognosis

  ○ Molecular profiling   - High
                                   - Likely responsiveness to purine analogue
                                   - Fludarabine (purine nucleoside analog)-based chemotherapy plus rituximab
                                   - Low likely response to purine nalaogues

  ○ Other immunotherapy

  ○ Transformation to   - R-CHOP
    large cell lymphoma

  ○ HSCT   - Curative, but ↑↑ risk of morbidity and mortality

➢ Complications

• Give 6 complications of CLL and its treatments.

  ○ Immune   - Hemolytic anemia
                                   - Thrombocytopenia

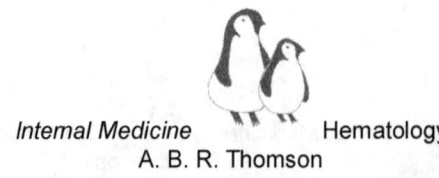

o Infection	- Pneumocystis jirovecii - CMV (Cytomegalovirus) - HSV (Herpes simplex virus)
o Blood disorders	- Hypogammaglobulinemia - Monoclonal gammapathies
o Transformation to	- Large cell lymphoma - Prolymphocytic leukemia

Hematopoietic Stem Cell Transplantation (HSCT)

➢ Types

  o Autologous

  o Allogenic

  - HLA-matched donor

  - Unrelated donor

➢ Preparative

  o ↑ CD_{34}^+ stem cells in circulation with G-CSF

  o Conditioning therapy for recipient

  - Myeloablative dose of cytotoxic chemotherapy, +/-

  - Whole body irradiation

  o Facilitate stem cell graft, and ↓ risk of CVHD (graft-versus-host disease) Immunosuppression

Hairy Cell Leukemia (HCL)

➢ Definition

  o Peripheral smear

  - Atypical lymphoid cells

  - Cytoplasmic projections giving lymphoid cells appearance of being "hairy"

  - CD11 and CD103 expression

  o Bone marrow

  - Fibrotic

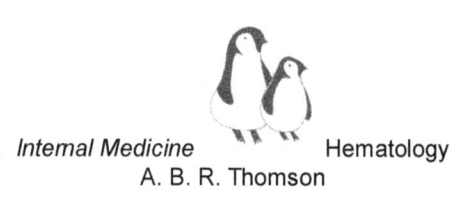

➢ Suspect in older men with

    o Cytopenia

    o Splenomegaly (no lymphadenopathy)

➢ Diagnosis

    o Bone marrow aspiration

    o Atypical lymphocytes with thread-like cytoplasmic projections from the surface of cells

    o Immunohistochemistry

➢ Treatment

    o Cladribine (parenteral purine analog)

CLINICAL GEM
Older, splenomegaly and pancytopenia but no lymphadenopathy-think of hairy cell leukemia. Think cladridine

---

➢ Diagnosis (peripheral smear)
    o Mature lymphocytes > 5000 / µL

    o "smudge" lymphocytes, distorted lymphocyte

    o B cell expression of CD19 and CD20

    o T cell expression of CD5

➢ Associated hematological changes
    o Hemolytic anemia (HA; direct Coombs positive warm autoantibody HA)

    o ITP (idiopathic thrombocytopenia)

    o Transformation
      - Large nodes, spleen, liver

➢ Therapy
    o Asymptomatic
      - Follow-up

    o Complicated
      - "B"-symptoms (e.g., fever, night sweats)
      - Advanced disease
      - Large tumor burden
      - Repeated infections

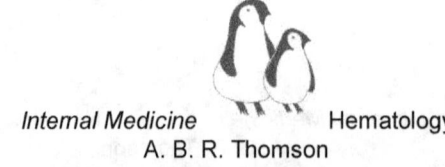

- o Drugs
  - Young
    - Fludarabine, cyclophosphamide plus rituximab
  - Older
    - Chlorambucil
- o HSCT
  - Resisting / relapsing CU
  - Transformation
- o Radiation
  - Painful lymphadenopathy
- o Splenectomy
  - Unresponsive
    - Cytopenia
    - Symptoms

Acute Lymphoblastic Leukemia / Lymphoma (ALL)

➢ Definition

- o ALL is a malignancy of B or T lymphocytes, with ≥ 25% lymphoblasts in bone marrow

➢ Causes
  - o Young age
  - o Aggressive disease precursors of T or B cells

➢ Clinical
  - o Bone marrow involvement → cytopenia
  - o CNS involvement
    - Common (30%)
  - o Mediastinum
    - Bulky nodes
  - o Less usual presentations

    - Anterior mediastinal mass
    - SVC (superior vena cava) syndrome
    - CNS involvement

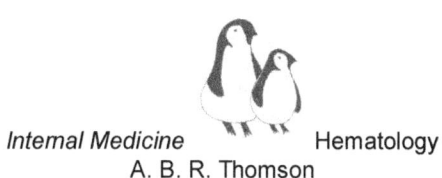

XXX

SO YOU WANT TO BE A HEMATOLOGIST!

- Give the physiological importance of the ↓ hepcidin concentration in iron deficiency.
  - When hepcidin is low, ferroportin in the duodenal enterocytes traffics to the basolateral membrane and facilitates the transfer of luminal (dietary) non-heme iron to the portal venous blood.
  - Also, in the presence of ↓ hepcidin, iron can be released from macrophages and used by the bone marrow for the production of erythrocytes.

The measurement of serum levels of vitamin B12 (cobalamin) do not reflect early deficiency in the body stores.

- Give 2 serum markers which reflect body stores and early deficiency of cobalamin.
  - ↑ homocysteine
  - ↑ MMA (methylmalonic acid)
  - Half marks for
    - ↑ LDH (lactate dehydrogenase)
    - ↑ Bilirubin

XXXXXXXXXXXXXXXXXXXXXXXXXXXXXXXXXXXXXXXXXXXXXXXXXXXXXXXXXXX

➢ Treatment
  - Induction chemotherapy plus HSCT
  - Bulky lymphadenopathy
    - Radiation
  - CNS prophylaxis
    - Intrathecal chemotherapy, +/- radiation

Acute Myeloid Leukemia (AML)

➢ Cause
  - Malignant clonal proliferation of myeloid cells
  - Primary
  - Secondary
    - Radiation
    - Chemotherapy
    - Benzene
    - Transformation
      - MPD (myeloproliferative disorder)
      - Myelodysplastic syndrome

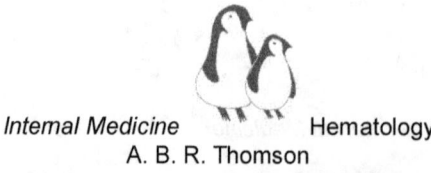

➢ Clinical

Pearl and Gem

- o Enlarged nodes, spleen and liver rarely occur in AMC
- o Common development of thrombocytopenia
- o Leukostasis syndrome
  - ↑↑↑ WBC (> 50,000 / μL) causes ↓ blood flow → tissue hypoxia
    - CNS
    - Lung
- o Tumor lysis syndrome treatment of AMC may be associated with ↑ release of cellular
  - K+
  - PO_4^-
  - Uric acid

➢ Diagnosis

- o Peripheral blood smear
  - ↑ WBC
  - ↓ RBC
  - ↓ platelets
  - ↑ Myeloblasts
    - CD34
    - HLA-DR
    - CD33
    - CD13
  - Auer rods. rod-shaped inclusion in myeloblast

- o Bone marrow
  - > 20% blasts
  - Cytogenetic studies
    - Prognosis
      - Good
      T(8;21), t(15;17), INV (16) or t (16;16)
      - Poor
      Loss / deletion of chromosome 7

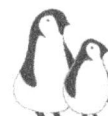

Punctuate translucencies in the skull vault are seen in persons with hyperparathyroidism.

- Give a systematic approach to the causes of mottling in the skull.

➤ Cancer
- o Metastases
- o Leukemia
- o Myeloma

➤ Hematological disorders
- o Sickle cell anemia
- o Histiocytosis X

➤ Endocrine disorders
- o Cushing disease
- o Hyperparathyroidism

➤ Treatment
- o IV fluids
- o Filtered and irradiated platelet transfusion for
  - Hemorrhage
  - Platelets < 10,000 / µL
- o Cytarabine and anthracycline
- o CD33+ AML- gemtuzumab ozogamicin (relapse older patients
- o t (15;17) translocation acute promyelocytic leukemia
  - ATRA (all-trans-retinoic acid)
- o Tumor lysis syndrome
  - Prevent
    Allopurinol plus rasburicase
  - Treat
    Hemodialysis for AKI (acute kidney injury)
- o Leukostasis syndrome
  - Leukapheresis

The t(15;17) translocation found on cytogenetic studies is associated with a good prognosis, but these patients with **acute promyelocytic leukemia** have an abnormal receptor for retinoic acid, which ↑ risk of fibrinolysis, DIC and bleeding.

- In the context of AML and acute promyelocytic leukemia, give the meaning of the **retinoic acid syndrome**.

  - o Patients with acute promyelocytic leukemia are treated with ATRA (all-transretinoic acid)
  - o ATRA may lead to
    - Fever
    - Lung symptoms
    - Hyperleukocytosis and leukostasis syndrome
    - Treat with dexamethasone

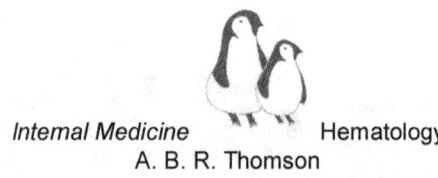

Internal Medicine   Hematology
A. B. R. Thomson

XXX

SO YOU WANT TO BE A HEMATOLOGIST!

- Give the differences between ALL and AML on cytochemical staining and flow cytometry.

Test	ALL	AML
Terminal deoxynucleotidyl transferase	+	-
Myeloperoxidase	-	+

- Give 3 cytogenetic changes in ALL that predict a poor prognosis.
  - Hypodiploidy
  - Translocations of MLL gene
  - Philadelphia chromosome (9;22)

Tumor lysis syndrome is common when ALL is treated with rasburicase.

- Give the reason why the patient should be tested for G-6-PD (glucose-6-phosphate dehydrogenase) deficiency before using rasburicase in ALL.
  - The patient with ALL plus G-6-PD deficiency given rasburicase may generate sufficient H_2O_2 (hydrogen peroxide) to develop hemolysis, or methemoglobinemia.
  - Because of the ↑ risk of CNS ALL, intrathecal chemoprophylaxis +/- cranial radiation is the standard of car
  - If ALL patient is positive for the Philadelphia chromosome, BCR-ABL inhibitors are given, plus cytotoxic chemotherapy

XXXXXXXXXXXXXXXXXXXXXXXXXXXXXXXXXXXXXXXXXXXXXXXXXXXXXXXXXXXXXXX

ATRA-induced differentiation Syndrome

➤ Definition
  - Treatment of patients with APL (acute promelocytic leukemia) with ATRA (all-trans-retinoic acid) or arsenic trioxide release cytokines from the differentiating promyelocytes, which cause capillary leakage in the lungs, resembling non-cardiac pulmonary edema.

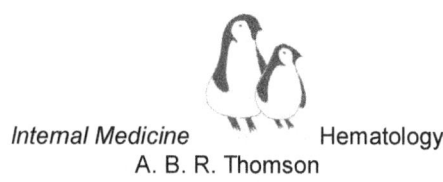

- ➤ Clinical
  - o Occurs in first (47%) or third (25%) weeks of treatment
  - o Symptoms and chest X-ray may suggest pulmonary infection, and antibiotics for possible pneumonia should be given with dexamethasone used to treat the ATRA-inducced differentiation syndrome

MKSAP Resource Site: www.mksap.acpontine.org

HEMATOLOGICAL MALIGNANCY

Lymphoma

- ➤ Types
  - o NHL   - Non-Hodgkin lymphoma B-I (85%), and NK-cell lymphomas
  - o HL   - Hodgkin lymphoma

- ➤ Associations

	NHL	HL
Immune suppression	++	+
HIV	Anaplastic large cell	
	Burkitt lymphoma	
HTLV-1	T cell	
HCV	B cell NHL, low-grade	
Drugs (immunosuppresants)	High-grade	
EBV	Burkitt	+
	PTLD	

  - o In a patient with treated HL, there is ↑ risk of NHL!

Abbreviations: EBV, Epstein-Barr virus; HIV, human immunodeficiency virus; HTLV, human T-cell lymphotropic virus type 1; PTLD, post-transplant lymphoproliferative disorder

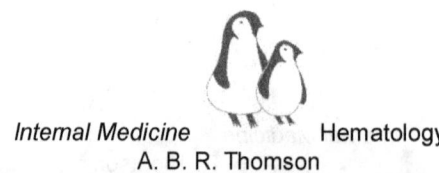

➢ Diagnosis
  ○ Exersional biopsy (**not** FNA [five needle aspiration])
  ○ Special testing of biopsy material
    - Histology
    - Molecular testing
      ▪ Cytogenetics
      ▪ FISH (fluorescence in situ hybridization)
      ▪ Gene expression profiling (immunohistochemistry)

➢ Staging and classification
  ○ Classification based on mature B cell, or mature T cell and NK cell, as well as numerous other factors
  ○ For the WHO (World Health Organization classification of Hodgkin and non-Hodgkin lymphomas, please see a standard textbook of medicine, UpToDate, or a recent review such as MKSAP 16, Hematology and Oncology, Table 43, page 99.
  ○ Phenotypes
    - B-cell
      Germinal centre, prognosis good
      Activated, prognosis
  ○ Prognostication
    - Indolent
    - Aggressive
    - Highly aggressive
  ○ Staging
    - Ann Arbor Staging System
    - IPI (International Prognostic Index) not routinely used anymore
    - FLIPI (Follicular Lymphoma International Prognostic Index)

Follicular Lymphoma

➢ Useful background
- o Accounts for
  - - 20% of all NHLs
  - - 70% of indolent NHLs
- o 90% have
  - - Rearrangements in Bcl-2 oncogene
  - - t (14;18) defect
- o Usually presents with advanced-stage disease, including bones marrow involvement
- o Treatment delayed until there are symptoms or organ dysfunction bone marrow lymph nodes

➢ Treatment options
- o Rituximab
- o R-CVP (rituximab plus cyclophosphamide)
- o R-CHOP (rituximab, cyclophosphamide, dororubicin, vincristine, prednisone)
- o Rituximab plus bendamustine
- o Tositumomab, horitumomab (radioimmunoconjugates)
- o HSCT
  - - Autologous
  - - Allogene

Abbreviation: HSCT, human stem cell transplantation

- • Give the name of the induction and maintenance therapy for indolent NHL (non-Hodgkin lymphoma, follicular lymphoma)

- o Chemotherapy plus rituximab
- o Low follicular lymphoma IPI (International Prognostic Index) – chemotherapy (cyclophosphamide, vincristine and prednisone) plus doxorubicin
- o High follicular lymphoma IPI – chemotherapy 9as above) plus rituximab

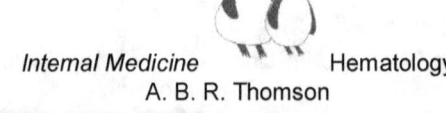

Internal Medicine   Hematology
A. B. R. Thomson

- o Note
  - - Radiotherapy may be used for maintenance but not for induction
  - - In the absence of symptoms, the patient is followed and not treated, regardless of the extent of the follicular lymphoma

Mantle Cell Lymphoma

➤ Definition

- o Overexpression of cyclin D1 and t(11;14) translocation on malignant lymphoid cells

➤ Presentation

- o Usually with stage IV disease involving
  - - Bone marrow
  - - Peripheral blood
  - - Small intestine
  - - Colon

➤ Diagnosis

- o Histopathology
- o Immunophenotyping
- o Immunohistochemistry
- o Cytogenetic testing

➤ Therapy

- o Assess therapeutic response with MIPI (Mantle cell International Prognostic Index)
- o Rituximab plus chemotherapy (R-HYPERCVAD)
- o HSCT
  - - Allogenic
  - - Autologous

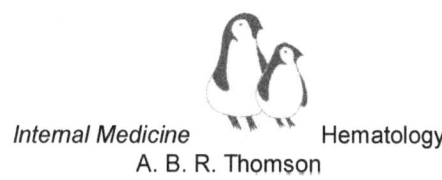

Hodgkin Lymphoma

➢ Treatment

    o Localized disease   Extended-field radiotherapy +/-
      chemotherapy

    o Advanced disease   ABVD (doxorubicin, bleomycin,
      vinblastine, dacarbazine)

    o CD20-positive lymphocyte predominant Hodgkin lymphoma R-ABVD
      (rituximab plus ABVD)

*poor prognosis factors

    o PET scan positive

    o Age > 45 yr

    o Males

    o Hemoglobin < 105 g/L (10.5 g/dL)

    o WBC > 15 x 10^9 /L (15,000 /µL)

Waldenstrom Macroglobulinemia (WM)

➢ Definition

    o Lymphoplasmacytic lymphoma (≥ 10% of bone marrow cellularity)
      characterized by production of monoclonal IgM antibodies

➢ Clinical

    o CNS

      - Peripheral sensorimotor neuropathy

      - ↑ anti-myelin glycoprotein antibodies

    o Blood

      - Platelet dysfunction

      - Anemia

      - Formation of Rouleaux

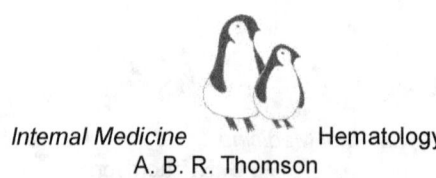

➢ Treatment

    ○ For symptoms WM plus ≥ 10% bone marrow lymphoplasmacytic involvement, or M protein ≥ 3 g/dL

      - Chemotherapy
         ▪ Rituximab (monoclonal anti-CD20 antibody, +/-
         ▪ Cytotoxic agent

          - Alkylating agent
             ▪ Chlorambucil
             ▪ Cyclophosphamide

          - Nucleoside
             ▪ Fludarabine
             ▪ Cladribine

Diffuse Large Cell Lymphoma

    ○ Most common type of NHL

    ○ B-cell diffuse NHL

      - R-CHOP +/- radiation

           ↓ relapse
         HSCT

    ○ T-cell NHL

      - CHOP

● Diffuse large cell lymphoma is the most common aggressive lymphoma. The initial chemotherapy is R-CHOP (rituximab plus cyclophosphamide, doxorubicin, vincristine and prednisone. Give the treatment of choice for the ~ 50% of patients who recur.

    ○ High dose R-CHOP, plus autologous HSCT

Mucosa-Associated Lymphoid Tissue (MALT) lymphoma

Useful background

    ○ B cells, CD20-positive

    ○ ~1/2 of all gastric lymphomas

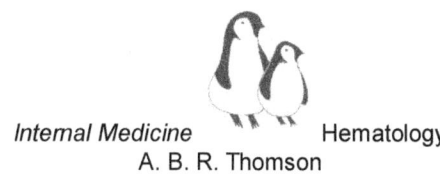

- o May be extranodal
  - Eye
  - Salivary glands
  - Thyroids
  - Lung
  - Colon
  - Bladder
- o May be limited to spleen, with no lymphadenopathy

➢ Associations

- o Helicobacter pylori infection
- o Autoimmune
  - Sjogren syndrome
  - Hashimoto thyroiditis

➢ Treatment

- o Triple therapy to eradicate H. pylori
- o Localized MALT
  - Radiation therapy
- o Advanced disease
  - Radiation plus rituximab, or
  - R-CVP (rituximab)
- o Splenectomy for MALT localized to spleen

Cutaneous T cell NHL

➢ Definition

- o T-cell which have
  - CD4 antigen
  - Large "cerebriform" nucleus
  - Clonal T-cell receptor

➢ Clinical

- o T-cell NHL of
  - Skin
    - Mycosis fungoides
  - Skin plus blood Sezary syndrome
- o Cell-mediated immunodeficiency, with
  - Recurrent bacterial infections
  - Sepsis

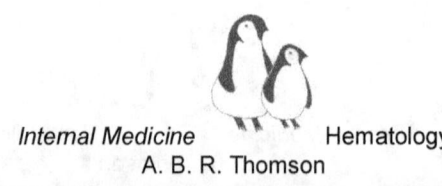

➢ Treatment
  o Early-stage-topical   - Topical   ▪ Corticosteroids and retinoids

         - PUVA   ▪ Psoralen and ultraviolet A light

  o Advanced   - Electron-beam radiation therapy, or
         - Extracorporeal photopheresis

  o Recalcitrant, or involving organs
         - CHOP
         - Alemtuzumab
         - HSCT, allogeneic

SPLENOMEGALY

➢ Definition
  o Hypersplenism
    - Reduction of 1 or more of the formed elements of the blood due to functional hyperactivity of the spleen

➢ Causes

• Give the causes of splenomegaly

  o Idiopathic

  o Infections
    - Viral: infective hepatitis, infectious mononucleosis
    - Bacterial: septicaemia, SBE, TB, syphilis brucellosis, typhoid
    - Rickettsial: typhus
    - Fungal: histoplasmosis
    - Protozoal: malaria*, kala-azar*, trypanosomiasis
    - Parasitic: hydatid cyst disease

  o Infiltration
    - Lymphoma
    - Leukemia (especially CML*)
    - Amyloid
    - Sarcoidosis
    - Gaucher, Nieman Pick disease
    - Benign tumors/ cysts
    - Myelofibrosis*

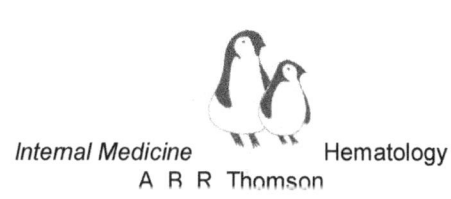

o Immune
- Rheumatoid arthritis (Felty syndrome)
- Systemic lupus erythematosis (SLE)

o Hematological
- Hemolytic anemia
- Myelofibrosis
- Polycythaemia rubra vera
- Occasionally in
  ▪ ITP
  ▪ Myelomatosis
  ▪ Megaloblastic anemia
  ▪ Chronic Fe-deficiency anemia

o Liver portal hypertension

o Endocrine
- Hyperthyroidism

*hugh spleen

Adapted from: Burton JL. *Churchill Livingstone* 1971, page 63; and Baliga RR. *Saunders/Elsevier* 2007, page 31.

➢ Clinical

• Clinical detection of splenomegaly

  o Several percent of the normal presumably healthy population may have palpable spleens. The "normal" spleen lies posterior to the left mid-axillary line, and between the 9th and 11th ribs. Normal dimensions are 3 x 7 x 12cm or less.

  o Because the spleen enlarges anteriorly and posteriorly, spleen size must increase by 40% before becoming palpable.

  o Only a small portion of the spleen protrudes beneath the costal margin, even when considerably enlarged.

  o Inspection should involve asking the patient to breath in deeply several times as well as looking at the "static" abdomen.

• Percussion in Traube Space and at Castell Spot

  o Traube's space is defined by the sixth rib superiorly, the left anterior axillary line laterally, and the costal margin inferiorly. Castell spot is located at the junction of the lowest intercostal space and the left

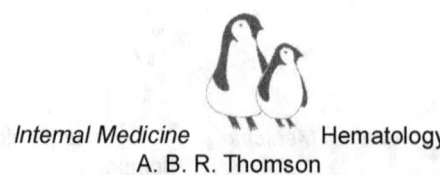

anterior axillary line. The value of Traube's space percussion (TSP) increases when combined with palpation.

○ Castell's sign: Percuss over the lowest intercostal space in the left anterior axillary line while asking the patient to inhale and exhale slowly and deeply. Resonance to percussion on expiration, replaced by dullness to percussion on inspiration suggests splenomegaly.

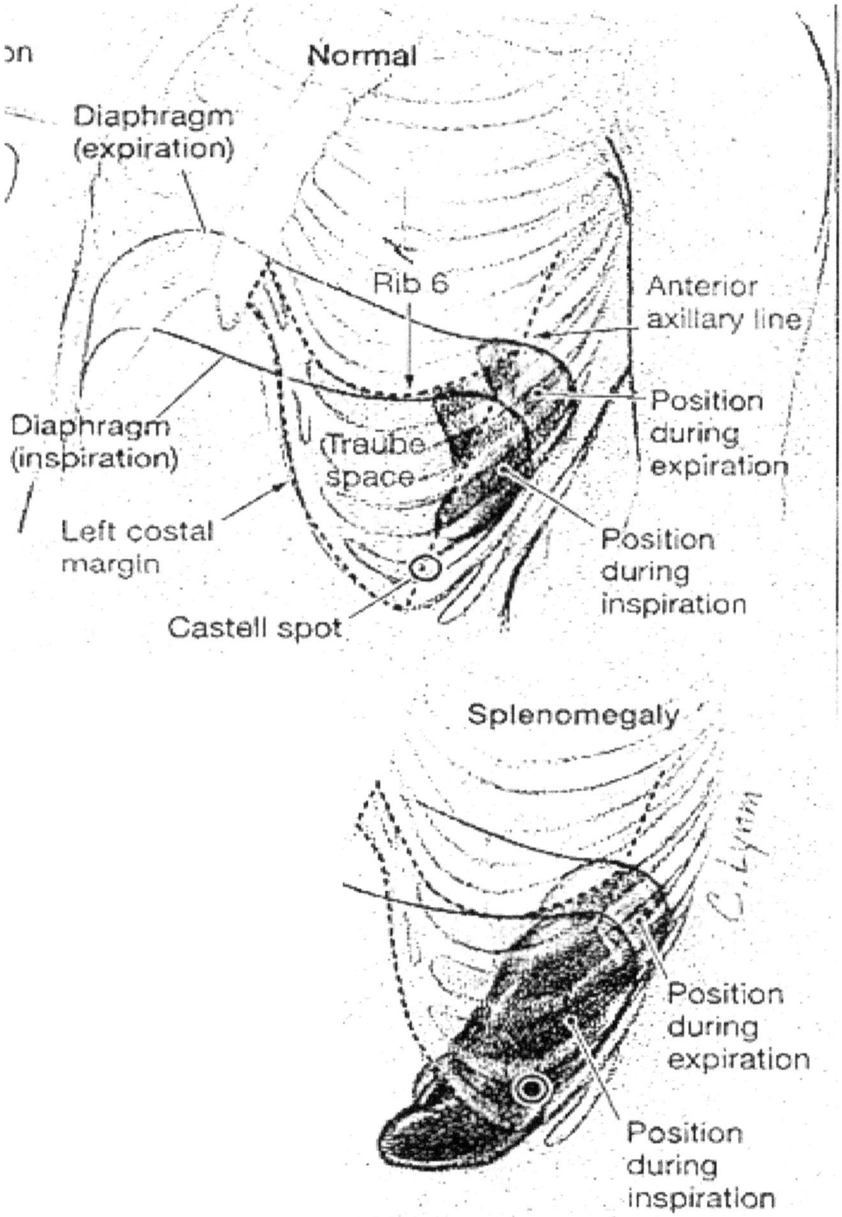

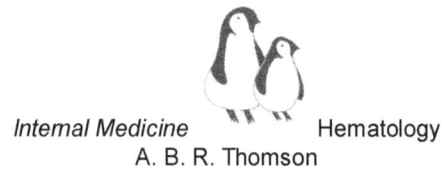

- Palpation

  o Percussion is more sensitive but less specific than palpation as a diagnostic test for splenomegaly.

  o Percussion (Castell's sign, Traube's space or Nixon method) should be done first, followed by palpation. If both percussion and palpation are positive, the diagnosis of splenomegaly can be ruled in, provided there is a pre-test probability of at least 10%.

  o Done with the patient supine, with the knees slightly flexed.

  o Start from the RLQ and work towards the LUQ, again assessing the effect of deep inspiration.

  o Remember that the left hand is not pulling the spleen forward to the right (examining) hand, but rather pulling the overlying skin forward to give enough slack for the right hand to properly feel under the costal margin.

  o Palpation is most useful in patients who have percussion dullness.

Nixon method to detect splenomegaly

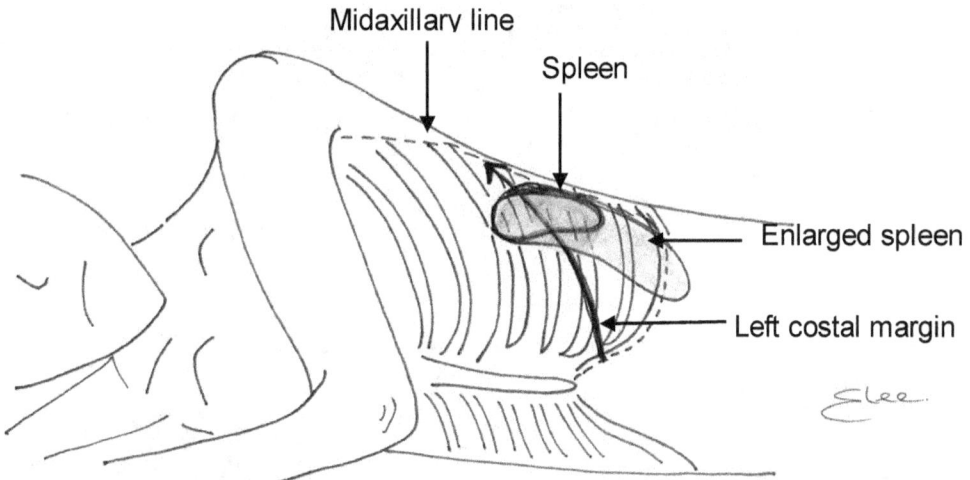

Positive indication: dullness is present more than 8 cm above the costal margin

  o Discriminate from other masses such as an enlarged kidney:
  - Feel for medial side splenic notching
  - The spleen moves towards the RLQ with inspiration, the kidney moves inferiorly

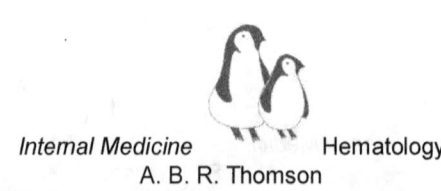

Internal Medicine   Hematology
A. B. R. Thomson

- Below the costal margin the relatively superficial spleen is dull to percussion; because of overlying bowel the enlarged kidney may sound resonant to percussion
- You cannot interpose your fingers between an enlarged spleen and the costal margin, it is however possible to palpate "above" a kidney.
- You may hear a "splenic rub".

Adapted from: Simel DL, et al. *McGraw-Hill Medical* 2009, Figure 46-3, page 607; Filate W, et al. *The Medical Society, Faculty of Medicine, University of Toronto* 2005, page 34; Davey P. *Wiley-Blackwell* 2006, pages 82 and 83.

- Give the factors which increase the pretest probability of finding splenomegaly.

  o Suspected or proven viral illness, lymphoproliferative disorder, or malignancy

  o Cirrhosis (portal hypertension)

  o Suspected or proven malaria

  o Connective tissue disorders associated with splenomegaly

Source: Simel DL, et al. *JAMA* 2009, page 613.

- Give the perform characteristics for detection of enlarged spleen.

Finding	PLR	NLR
o Palpation	8.5	0.5
o Percussion	**6.5**	0.2
- Nixon method	2.0	0.7
- Traube space dullness	2.1	0.8

Abbreviation: NS, not significant; NLR, negative likelihood ratio; PLR, positive likelihood ratio; MCL, midclavicular line

NLR	Probability	PLR	
	Decrease		Increase

-45%	-30%	-15%		+15%	+30%	+45%	
0.1	0.2	0.5	1	2	5	10	

LRs

Note that the Castell sign has a PLR < 2, and is not included here. Also, the spleen examination has a low sensitivity, especially if the pre test probability for splenomegaly is < 10%.

Abbreviation: NLR, negative likelihood ratio; PLR, positive likelihood ratio

Adapted from: McGee SR. *Saunders/Elsevier* 2007, Box 47.1, page 554.

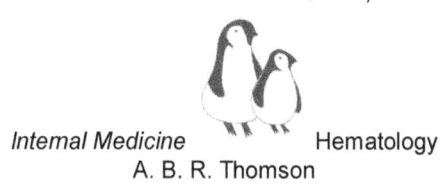

Internal Medicine   Hematology
A. B. R. Thomson

Useful background: Performance characteristics for palpation of spleen in various disorders

- o Palpable spleen in returning travelers with fever, detecting malaria
- o Palpable spleen in patients with non-obstructive jaundice, detecting hepatocellular disease
- o Palpable spleen in patients with chronic liver disease, detecting cirrhosis
- o Note
  - The likelihood of a high PLR for splenomegaly depends on the clinical setting
  - For example
    - In a returning traveler and fever where there is splenomegaly from malaria (PLR,6.6)
    - Much lower values to detect hepatocellular disease in a person with non-obstructive jaundice (2.9), or detecting cirrhosis in the person with chronic liver disease (2.3).

Abbreviation: likelihood ratio (LR) if finding present = positive LR (PLR)

Adapted from: McGee SR. *Saunders/Elsevier* 2007, Box 47.2, pages 556 -7.

SO YOU WANT TO BE A HEMATOLOGIST!

- Percussion in Traube space is not specific for splenomegaly. Give what other conditions cause dullness here.

  - o Left pleural effusion
  - o Large pericardial effusion
  - o Massive cardiomegaly
  - o Stomach full of food
  - o Splenic flexure of colon full of feces
  - o Enlarged left kidney

Splenomegaly accompanies hepatomegaly in persons with portal hypertension.

- Give the exceptions to this clinical "rule"?
  - o Congenital asplenia
  - o Post-surgical asplenia
  - o Splenic vein thrombosis
  - o Multiple splenic vein infarctions

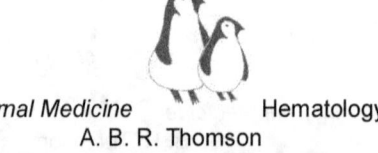

Internal Medicine   Hematology
A. B. R. Thomson

Amyloidosis (AL; immunoglobulin light-chain amyloidosis)

➢ Definition

  o β-pleated sheets of protein fibrils of λ and κ monoclonal light chains causing end-organ damage, and associated with multiple myeloma in ~ 10%

➢ Clinical

  o Major sites of deposit of light chains

   - CNS / PNS
     ▪ Distal sensorimotor neuropathy
     ▪ Autonomic neuropathy
     ▪ Carpal tunnel syndrome

   - CVS
     ▪ Restrictive cardiomyopathy
     ▪ Interventricular septal hypertrophy

   - GI
     ▪ GI tract infiltration
       - Hepatomegaly
       - Macroglossia

   - Kidney
     ▪ Nephrotic syndrome

➢ Diagnosis

  o Protein electrophoresis and immunofixation
  o IgG lambda M protein
   - Serum
   - Urine
  o Free light chains

➢ Biopsy pathology

  o Affected organ
  o Combination of fat pad plus bone marrow biopsy
  o Amorphous eosinophilic amyloid protein deposits
  o Apple-green birefringence with Congo red stain examined under polarized light
  o IF / IHC deposits of clonal chains

Abbreviations: IF, immunofluorescence; IHC, immunohistochemistry

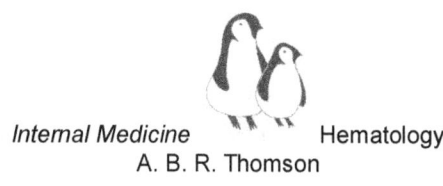

Internal Medicine   Hematology
A. B. R. Thomson

➢ Treatment

   o Melphalan plus dexamethasone

   o Autologous HSCT (less effective than in MM)

SO YOU WANT TO BE A HEMATOLOGIST!

- Perform a focused physical examination of the head and neck for AL amyloidosis.
  - o Eyes – "Racoon eyes" from periorbital ecchymosis
  - o Macroglossia

- Give the name of serological markers for cardiac involvement in AL amyloidosis which are predictive of mortality (median overall survival).
  - o Troponin T
  - o N-terminal pro-B-type naturetic peptide

Number of positive serological markers	Median overall survival, mon
0	26
1	11
2	4

HEMATOLOGY AND PREGNANCY

To be considered here

   o Gestational anemia

   o Sickle cell disease

   o Gestational thrombocytopenia

   o Immune thrombocytopenic purpura

   o Microangiopathy of pregnancy

   o Thromboembolism in pregnancy

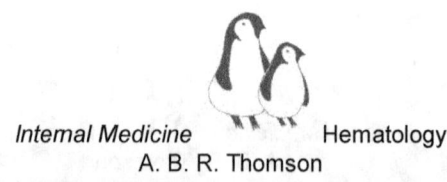

Gestational Anemia

Physiological anemia of pregnancy

- ↑ erythropoietin → ↑ RBC mass ⎤
- ↑↑ plasma volume → ↓ blood viscosity ⎬ → ↑ O2 carrying
- ↑iron requirements for ↑ RBC mass and for fetus ⎦
- Parenteral iron in pregnancy

Product	FDA class
Iron dextran	C (presumed uncertain)
Iron sucrose, ferric gluconate	B (presumed safe)

- ↑ folate
  - Requirements for ↑ RBC mass and for fetus
  - To prevent neural tube defects

Sickle Cell Disease in Pregnancy

- Hydroxyurea **not** to be used in pregnancy
  - Stop at least 3 mon before pregnancy-related planned conception
- Team approach because of ↑ mortality for
  - Homozygous SS ~ 2%
  - Compound heterozygotes (5 plus B-thalassemia or HbC) ~ 1% trait – normal complication rate
- Complications
  - ↑ mortality
  - Menarche later
  - First pregnancy later
  - ↑ fetal loss
  - ↑ number of low-birth weight neonates

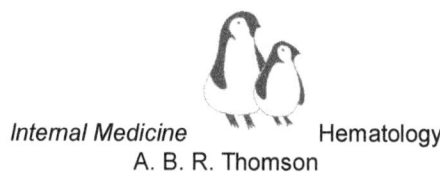

➢ Treatment
  o Vaginal delivery
  o For pain
    - Opioids (but not Demerol / Meperidine)
  o For severe anemia plus HF (heart failure)
    - Transfusion
  o And say it again
    - **No** hydroxyurea (teratogenic)

• Give the reason why meperidine is not a first choice analgesics.

  o Meperidine is metabolized to normeperidine
  o Normaperidine accumulates as a toxic metabolite
  o Normeperidine lowers the seizure threshold

Thrombocytopenia in Pregnancy

Treatment target
  o When to give platelets in pregnancy
    - Asymptomatic, Pl < 50,000 / μL
    - Symptomatic, < 30 – 40,000 / μL
    - Cesarean section, < 50,000 / μL
    - Neuraxial anesthesia, < 80,000 / μL
  o Thrombocytopenia in neonate
    - Anti-platelet antibodies may cross the placenta
    - Thrombocytopenia in neonate ~ 10%
    - Problems with measuring fetal platelet levels
      Scalp vein sampling is misleading
      Umbilical cord sampling may cause miscarriage (1%)

Gestational Thrombocytopenia in Pregnancy

- o A "physiological" effect of pregnancy, due to
    - ↑ blood volume → dilutional thrombocytopenia
- o Suspect pathological cause of thrombocytopenia
    - If platelets < 50 x 10^9 / L (50,000 /μL
    - If ↓ platelets in T1 or T2 (first or second terms)

Immune Thrombocytopenic Purpura (ITP) in Pregnancy

- o ITP may
- o ITP is a diagnosis of exclusion: for thrombocytopenia occurring in pregnancy, consider
    - Gestational thrombocytopenia
    - Preeclampsia
    - HELLP
    - DIC
    - TTP

Abbreviations: HELLP, hemolysis elevated liver enzymes low platelet count; DIC, disseminated intravascular coagulation

Microangiopathy In Pregnancy

C	T1	T2	T3	Postpartum
	← TTP – HUS →		Preeclampsia	preeclampsia
	↓		↓ ~ 10%	
	MAHA		HELLP	
	Thrombocytopenia		AFLP	
	↓		↓	
	PE		Delivery	

Abbreviation: AFLP, acute fatty liver of pregnancy; C, conception; HELLP, hemolysis elevated liver enzymes low platelet count; HUS, hemolytic uremic syndrome; MAHA, microangiopathic hemolytic anemia; T, trimester; TTP, thrombotic thrombocytopenic purpura;

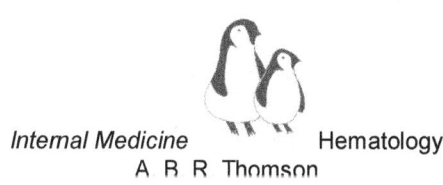

Trying to Keep Things Straight re Complications in Pregnancy

	MAHA	↓ platelets	PT/aPTT	DIC	↓ BS	↑ SBP	Proteinuria	LE
o Preeclampsia	-	-	-	-	-	+	+	↑ AT
o HELLP	+	+	N	-	-	+/-	+	+
o TTP-HUS	+	+	-	-	-	-	-	-
o AFLP	-	-	↑	+	+	-	-	↑ Ch

Abbreviations: AFLP, acute fatty liver of pregnancy; aPTT, activated partial thromboplastin time; Ch, cholestatic liver tests; DIC, disseminated intravascular coagulation; HELLP, hemolysis elevated liver enzymes low platelet count; HUS, hemolytic uremic syndrome; MAHA, microangiopathic hemolytic anemia; PT, prothrombin time; TTP, thrombotic thrombocytopenic purpura

CLINICAL CLUES

- o Preeclampsia
  - Half occur T3, ~ half post-partum
  - 10% progress to HELLP
- o HELLP
  - Half have hypertension
  - Half are normotensive

"Don't judge each day by the harvest you reap but by the seeds you plant"
Robert Louis Stevenson

Thromboembolism in Pregnancy

- o ↑↑↑ risk of VTE 1 to 6 week post-partum

- Give the management of the pregnant patient with suspected VTE (venothromboembolism).

  - o Stratify risk

↑ odds ratio	Condition	
↑↑↑↑ (25x)	Previous VTE	(Venothromboembolism)
↑↑↑ (7-8x)	SLE	(systemic lupus erythmatosis)
	SCA	(sickle cell anemia)
	HD	(heart disease)
↑↑ (4x)	↑ BMI	(obesity)
↑ (2x)	Anemia	
	↑ age > 35 year	
	DM	(diabetes mellitus)
	↑ BP	(hypertension)

- ➢ Diagnosis
  - o DCUS (duplex compression ultrasonography) if DCUS negative

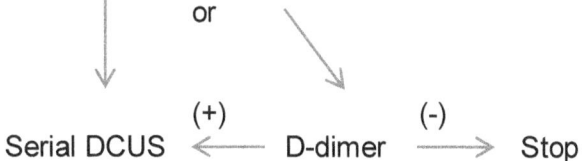

      or

                              (+)   (-)
      Serial DCUS ⟵——— D-dimer ———⟶ Stop

  - o MRI venography
    - - For IVC (inferior vena cava)
  - o V/Q (ventilation / perfusion) scan
  - o CTA (CT angiography), abdominal shielding

- ➢ Treatment
  - o VTE in

    Month 0-8   LMWH

    Month 9   UFH (can easily be reversed peridelivery)

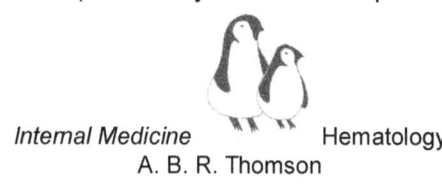

- o VC (vena cava) filter
- o Warfarin
  - During (3-6 mon) / after pregnancy (6 to 12 week)

    Okay to use warfarin with nursing

- Give the optimum time to screen a patient with VTE for a thrombophilia disorder.

  - o It is controversial whether patients should be tested for thrombophilia, but if such testing is done, it should be performed months after the acute event and when warfarin has been stopped

- Give the management of the patient with an INR of 1.2 when tested 2 weeks after hospital discharge for VTE.

  - o The INR is subtherapeutic, the risk of repeat VTE is high (40% in first month after VTE id not properly anti-coagulated, and the INR will not be corrected for 3 days after the appropriate ↑ dose of warfarin

  - o For these reasons, give LMWH while frequently ↑ warfarin to correct the INR

IMMUNOGLOBULIN DEFICIENCY

➢ Causes

- Give a systematic approach to the causes of immunoglobulin deficiency.

  - o Primary
    - Physiological (in infancy)
    - Congenital sex-linked (Bruton)
    - A lymphocytic (Swiss)
    - Lymphopenic (Gitlin)
    - Associated with thymoma (Goods)
    - Associated with thrombocytopenia and eczema (Wiskott-Aldrich)
    - Ataxia telangiectasia (Louis-Bar)

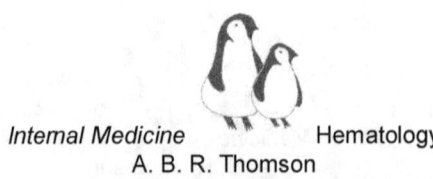

Internal Medicine Hematology
A. B. R. Thomson

- o Secondary
  - Protein deficiency
  - ↓ synthesis
    - Leukemia
    - Lymphoma
    - Myeloma
    - Waldenstrom's macroglobulinemia
    - Irradiation
    - Cytotoxic drugs

➢ Pathophysiology

- In the adult, a deficiency of serum immunoglobulins may be the result of protein deficiency, hypercatabolic states, or from decreased synthesis resulting from bone marrow disorders, reticuloendothelial neoplasia, or toxic factors. Give 10 causes of secondary immunoglobulin deficiency.

  - o ↓ intake of protein

  - o ↓ absorption
    - Malabsorption e.g. celiac disease
    - Protein – leasing enteropathy

  - o ↑ loss
    - Nephritic syndrome
    - Burns
    - Extensive dermatitis
    - Pulmonary loss

  - o ↓ use
    - Hypercatabolic state

  - o ↓ synthesis
    - Marrow disorders
      - Metastases
      - Myelosclerosis
      - Hypoplasia
      - Leukemia
      - Lymphoma
      - Myeloma
      - Macroglobulinemia
      - Hodgkin disease

  - o "toxic" factors
    - Irradiation
    - Diabetes
    - Thyrotoxicosis
    - Sepsis
    - Steroids, cytotoxic drugs

*Note: Any of the above factors may worsen a primary immunoglobulin deficiency.

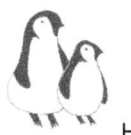

Internal Medicine   Hematology
A. B. R. Thomson

- Macroglobulinemia occurs in Waldenstrom macroglobulinemia (WM) as well as in multiple myeloma (MM). What complications of MM are rare in WM?

  o Kidney
    - Chronic renal failure

  o Bone
    - Hypercalcemia
    - Osteolytic bone lesions
    - Amyloidosis

➢ Clinical

  o When to suspect

    - Infections
      - Frequent
      - Multiple
      - Prolonged

    - Often due to
      - Streptococcus pneumonia
      - Haemophilus influenza
      - Neisseria

    - Consequence
      - Often asymptomatic
      - Infection giardia lamblia
      - Inflammation / infection
      - False-negative anti-IgA e.g. anti-tissue transglutaminase (to diagnose celiac disease)
      - Anaphylactic transfusion reaction (from anti-IgA antibodies developed in transfusion recipient)

- In the context of serum immunoglobulins, what are the features of Waldenstrom macroglobulinemia, and what are the causes of an M band?

➢ Definition

  o An M band is an increase in serum IgG, IgA or IgM occurring as the result of the increase in one clone of cells to produce increased amounts of only one immunoglobulin

  o The one clonal production of increased amounts of immunoglobulin is called "monoclonal gammopathy"

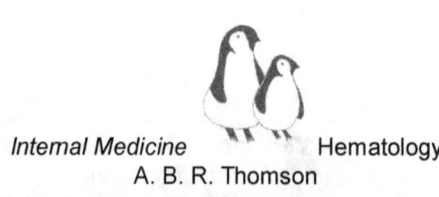

- o Waldenstrom
  - - Hepatosplenomegaly
  - - Lymphadenopathy
  - - Anemia
  - - Coagulopathy
  - - ↑ macroglobulins
  - - ↑ blood viscosity
    - ▪ Organ ischemia (e.g. CHF, SOB, retinal bleeding, paresis, neuropathies, myelopathies)

- ➢ Causes
  - o Idiopathic
  - o Myeloma
  - o Bence Jones proteinuria without myeloma
  - o Heavy chain disease
  - o Leukemia, lymphoma, carcinoma

Selective IgA Deficiency

- ➢ Demography
  - o Autosomal
    - - Recessive, or
    - - Dominant, with incomplete penetrance
  - o ~ 1:500 persons

- ➢ Clinical
  - o Recurrent infections
    - - Pulmonary
    - - GI giardiasis
    - - GU UTI
  - o Autoimmune disorders e.g. celiac disease
  - o Atopic disorders
  - o Anaphylaxis when given
    - - Immunoglobulin
    - - Blood products

- ➢ Laboratory
  - o ↓↓ IgA

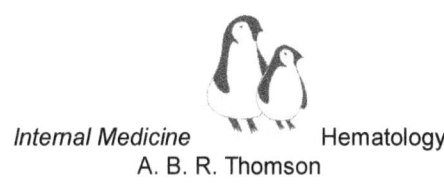

o May also have
  - ↓ IgG2
  - ↓ IgM

o Autoantibodies to IgA

CLINICAL CAUTION

• Give the reason why persons with undetectable serum levels of IgA are at risk of transfusion reactions or anaphylaxis when given preparations of immune globulin.
  o Persons with selective IgA deficiency may form antibodies directed against IgA, which places the patient at risk for blood transfusion of IV immunoglobulins

---

Common Variable Immunodeficiency (CVID)

➢ Cause
  o ↓ B cell differentiation
    - ↓ production of immunoglobulins (↓↓ IgG, ↓ IgA, ↓ IgM)

➢ Clinical
  o Ear, sinuses, eye
    - Infection

  o Lung
    - Bronchiectasis
    - COPD
    - CRPD (chronic restrictive pulmonary disease)

  o GI
    - Candida
    - Giardia lamblia
    - Enteroviruses
    - IDD
    - Celiac disease

  o MSK
    - RA (rheumatoid arthritis)

  o Blood
    - Hemolytic anemia
    - Thrombocytopenia
    - PA (pernicious anemia)

  o Miscellaneous
    - Non-caseating granulomas
    - ↓ response to (protein or polysaccharide based)

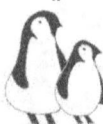

➢ Treatment   o Antibiotic prophylacxis

     o Associated chronic infections

     o Use of > 1 mon
- Corticosteroids
- Immunosuppressants

     o Immunoglobulins

- Give the common clinical presentations of CVI (common variable immunodeficiency).

     o Lung   - Sinopulmonary infections

     o GI   - Malbasorption

     o Autoimmune disorders

     o Lymphoma

Complement System

➢ Inherited usually   o Autosomal recessive; except
     o Autosomal dominant C1 inhibition deficiency
     o X-linked properdin deficiency

➢ Acquired

➢ Clinical   o ↑ risk of infections
     o Streptococcus pneumonia (encapsulated pneumonia)
- 3, H, I, properdin
- Neisseria meningococcus, N. gonococcus
- Properdin
  - Neissera
  - Recurrent
    - Pneumonia
    - Otitis media
     o ↑ risk of SLE and other autoimmune disorders
↓ C1, C2, C3, C4

➢ Diagnosis   o Test for CH_{50} (total hemolytic complement), their specific components

➢ Treatment   o Routine conjugate vaccine

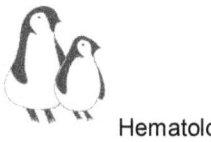

INDEX

Note: Page number followed by f and t indicates figure and table respectively.

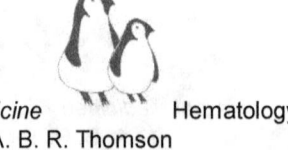

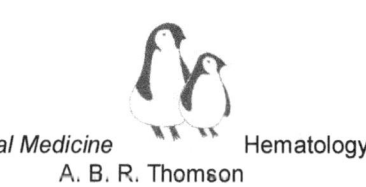

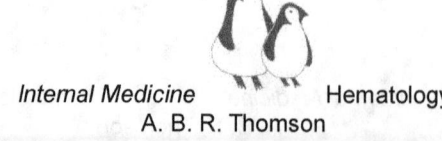

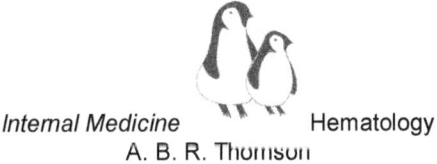

treatment, 69
Essential thrombocythemia, 59–61
   bleeding disorder in, 60
   clinical, 60
   definition, 59–60
   laboratory, 60
   treatment, 61

F
Factor V Leiden (FVL), 6–7
Febrile neutropenia, 51, 110
Febrile non-hemolytic transfusion reaction, 46
FFP. *See* Fresh frozen plasma
Fluorescence in situ hybridization testing, for CML, 59
Follicular lymphoma, 124–125
   background, 124
   treatment options, 124–125
Fondaparinux, for venothrombotic embolism, 17
Fresh frozen plasma (FFP), 43
FVL. *See* Factor V Leiden

G
Gestational anemia, 137
Gestational thrombocytopenia, 29–30, 29t, 30t
Glucose-6-phosphate dehydrogenase (G-6-PD) deficiency, 96, 102

H
Hairy cell leukemia (HCL), 115–117
   definition, 115
   diagnosis, 116
   hematological changes, 116
   older men with, 116
   peripheral smear (diagnosis), 116
   therapy for, 116–167
   treatment, 116
HCL. *See* Hairy cell leukemia
Heinz bodies, 80
Hematological malignancy, 122–129
   cutaneous T cell NHL, 128–129
      clinical, 128
      definition, 128
      treatment, 129
   diffuse large cell lymphoma, 127
   follicular lymphoma, 124–125
      background, 124

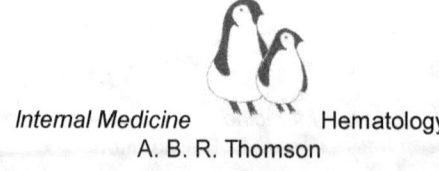

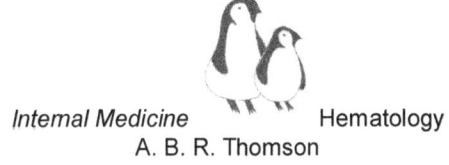

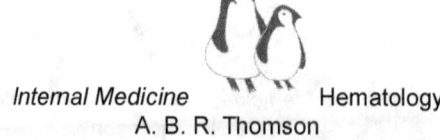

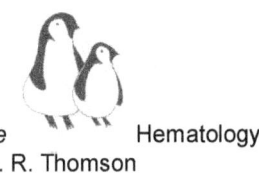

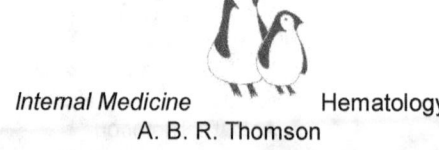

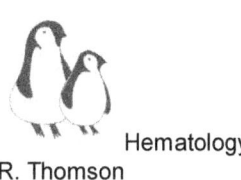

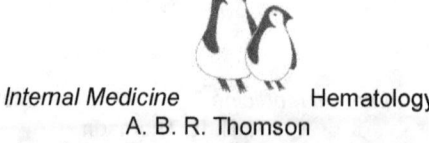

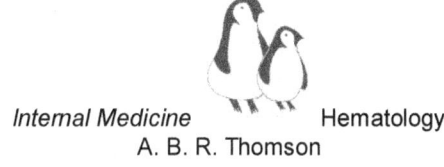

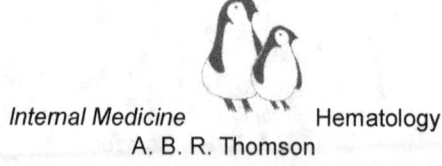

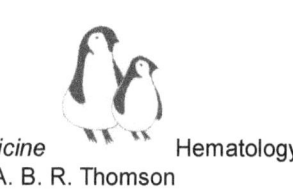

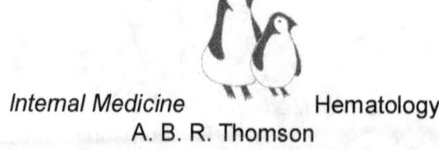